WORLD KEYS TO **HEALTH** *&LONG LIFE*

i

DEDICATION

I dedicate this book to two wonderful men whom I have been privileged to know in this life, and to a country that has inspired me to gather the survival principles in human beings leading to a healthy long life.

The countries we visited with these men have shown me that survival is an underlying principle for good health and for the prolongation of life. These two men brought me in contact with the people there.

The first man, Mr. Peter Maloff, was a man of peace, a man of deep convictions and one who had a deeply-earnest motivation to bring about the survival of mankind by ending war and helping others to live a higher and better life. He was a vegetarian of three generations and a Doukhobor, living the simple life in British Columbia, Canada.

The second man, Mr. Vahab Chazarian, made it possible for me to be in touch with those who had to consider survival a necessity. I am indebted to the country to which he introduced me, a country that has gone through much strife, mental oppression and the hatreds of war.

Yet, in spite of it, this country demonstrated more love and generosity to me on my visit than any other; and it gave me the feeling that the people there have overcome and are emerging and moving to the top, carrying with them their culture, ideals and beliefs. This is the only country in the world that decided to go all out in uniting together with the bonds of Christian faith, each and everyone. This was a demonstration of how unity of ideals and individual compassion for their country enabled the people to survive.

I dedicate this book to these two men and to the country of Armenia.

While we have spent our last years in seeking out longevity principles in people, it is the Spirit of Survival—physical, mental and spiritual—which is the dominant factor for long life and good health.

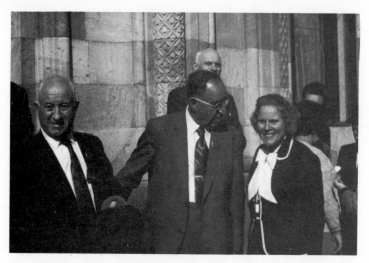

Mr. Vahan Ghazarian, his associate, my wife, Marie, and Mr. Peter Maloff in the background. Taken in front of the Hotel Erevan in Erevan, Armenia.

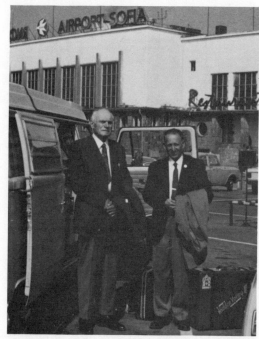

Dr. Jensen and Mr. Peter Maloff leaving Turkey on their way to Bulgaria.

WORLD KEYS TO HEALTH & LONG LIFE

by Bernard Jensen

BiWorld Publishers Inc.

A division of Amtec

P.O. Box 62 Provo, Utah 84601

Library of Congress Catalog Card Number
75-9184

ISBN 0-89127-107-4

Printed in the U.S.A. by

Microlith Printing Inc.

A division of Amtec

Introduction

I SEARCH FOR WORLD KEYS

This book has been compiled with one idea in mind: One picture is worth a thousand words, and maybe 10,000 words!

Volumes and volumes could be written on variations of these Keys, and could be expanded ad infinitum; so we have coordinated thoughts that could help you in your search for a good life and a long one.

It is not enough to just have a good physical body without a balanced brain. There are faculties of the mind which must be fed and expressed. A person must be happy to be well and be well to be happy. When a man jumps for joy, he should have the body with which to jump. On the other hand, he cannot expect sweet thoughts with a sour stomach.

Our travels confirmed our teachings of living the natural life; and our teachings, in turn, were influenced by our travels.

It was a joy to see these old people, living in balance with nature: eating the proper foods, living at the right altitude in a good climate, practicing the art of love and strong family ties, unaware that they held the Keys to good health and therefore to a long life.

All of life should be integrated—spiritual, mental and physical. The same ideas and ideals have come up again and again in my practice of the past 48 years, and we welcome this opportunity to share them with you.

Each country had something to contribute towards the prolongation of life and survival.

Consider and study:

In JAPAN, iodine from seafood was used so much in

their diet that there was very little goiter, but in SWITZER-
LAND many people in the mountains had this disease
because of the lack of iodine. It was in these countries
that we could see the effects of environment upon the
body.

FIJI ISLANDERS had iron in their diets, but not the calcium. NEW ZEALAND gives us the rest, relaxation and
recreation principle. The lack of protein in INDIA is a
known fact among nutritionists and has its effect upon the
whole country.

The BRITISH sailor of the past was called "limey" because he traveled with so many of the fruit aboard ship for
the prevention of scurvy. In PERU people living at altitudes of 10,000 feet would have a blood count of 7,500,000,
while at the ocean it is very difficult to find anyone with
a blood count above 5,000,000. This shows the relationship of altitude to our good health.

The philosophy of CHINA and the spirituality of
ARMENIA shows the mental needs of a person for good
health. The calcium and the strength of the TURKS shows
their need for this element.

It is in the relationship to our environment—how we
live, whether it be in our mind or deeds—that determines
whether we live the long life or not.

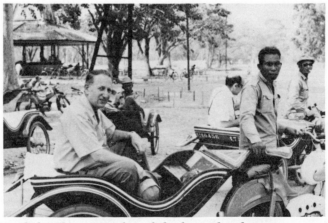

My search for the principles of the keys that keep a person well
and contribute to his long life, is one which has taken us many
years and through many countries. Through joining me in my
search, may good health and long life be yours.

Table of Contents

Table of Contents (continued)

Table of Contents (continued)

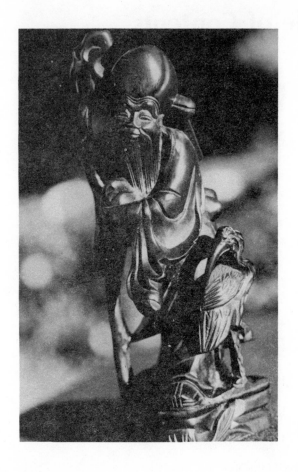

In Chinese mythology, the God of Longevity is one of the eight immortals. Immortality has been the object of man's search since time immemorial. Thus spirituality and a philosophy developed. The peach held in the hand of this statue symbolizes man's earthly needs. The staff on which he leans symbolizes spirituality. The two united betoken good health and a long life.

Chapter 1

SENSELESS SENILITY

Man has sought the elixir of life and has pursued the vague promise of lasting youth or immortality since the beginning of time. My search along these lines has caused numerous theories to come to my attention. The Keys to the well-guarded secrets of longevity may well turn out to be a combination of interacting causes. Emotional poise, balanced nutrition and favorable environment are just some of the basic elements of a long and satisfying life. No one isolated item can suffice in maintaining perfect health. We must pursue an intelligent course of action which is possible only through a better knowledge of what our bodies need.

Yes, the need of the hour is to learn what all these factors are so that we no longer commit needless offenses on our poor defenseless bodies. It was this very thirst for more and more knowledge on the subject of longevity that led me to my world-wide travels in search of definite answers to the many questions mankind have wrestled with for so long. Each of us needs to embark on a similar course of study, and this book has been prepared to enable you to initiate your own search and draw your own conclusions. Once we accept the premise that senility is senseless and not inevitable, we can apply ourselves to the task of learning what we need to avoid, as well as what we should try to attain.

Gerontology, or the study of the aging process, is a fairly recent pursuit of the intellectual and scientific community. The pathological causes for aging are slowly becoming apparent. These detrimental elements which slowly and inexorably rob us of our youth need to be pinpointed and, if possible, eliminated to some extent from our experience. On the positive and encouraging side is the theory that the human body has the inherent ability to renew itself indefinitely. This theory is gaining wider and wider acceptance and is being substantiated by countless experiments on animals and to a lesser extent among humans.

Life presents many problems. We all have them. It would seem then that one of our most basic needs is to attain harmony. Man needs contentment and a sense of peace. Financial worries, a disagreeable job, an incompatible marriage and resentment are all slow killers. These things interfere with our bodily functions just as certainly as do the poor eating habits we may have. Man has to be in harmony with all that exists before he can get well. Even though he possesses all of the chemistry for regenerating the cell structure in his body, yet without harmony all these wonderful physical attributes could be destroyed in a short time.

The dictionary definition of health is hale, or whole. The body is as good as the weakest organ, just as every chain is as strong as its weakest link. In other words, when the body begins to age, or deteriorate, and some one organ begins to break down, we find that the whole body is breaking down with it. We hear of scientists who try to inject glandular substances into bodies for rejuvenation purposes. We hear of them trying to put young glands of monkeys or goats into old bodies in the effort to rejuvenate them, but these old bodies were so broken down they could not support these new gland structures. That is why it is important to realize that the whole body must be taken into consideration. In the future, it will be recognized that this body must be treated in its "wholeistic" sense rather than just in parts and there must be a combination of Keys that reach every cell in the body and motivate the life force within to prevent senility.

As an example, there was the case of Mr. Blaiberg in South Africa. He lived for nearly two years with a transplanted heart. Upon reading his diary we learn that he spent as much as six hours a day just preparing himself to go outside to talk to a reporter or to tell someone about his condition. An interesting point is that he didn't die of heart trouble, but of six other ailments. This bears out the fact that it is important to consider the body as a whole, rather than seeking health by doctoring one small part.

THE VITAL LIFE FORCE

I wonder if we can ever really know what life is. We do know that life must include energy and vitality. Life in the body seems to depend in part on the harmonious functioning of the endocrine glands and the intestinal tract. We need to realize that we deprive the body of its life forces when we do not eat properly. Good nutrition is an important essential in order that the organs may work in perfect harmony with each other.

In some of the Keys, we learn that the aging process may be dependent upon how well the brain is cared for and the amount of activity in which a person engages. The brain could be considered the motor of the body and there must be a proper amount of cerebral blood flowing to the mind, for every organ in the body depends upon the brain action. It is not only the quality of the blood that is important, but the amount of blood that gets to the brain. This is the reason why there is so much emphasis in the Keys on Circulation and Exercise on the importance of keeping the legs in good condition. We noticed that all the elderly people we met were busy people. Their days were filled with activity. We also noticed particularly that none of these old people were made to feel useless, unwanted, or burdensome.

The mind can be capable of exerting either a negative or a positive influence on the body. We know, for instance, that during a hypnotic experiment, it is possible for a man who might ordinarily be able to lift only 125 pounds, yet under hypnosis, this same man could lift as much as 300 to 400 pounds. I have seen people in the Fiji Islands walk on the hottest coals and stones, and come out unharmed, with no tissue damage whatsover. Similar experiments have been performed with people under hypnosis in which lighted cigarette butts pressed into the palm of the hand failed to produce a burn when the individual was made to believe he would not be harmed. It makes one aware that there must be an important connection between the brain cells and the well-being of all other bodily cells. Our emotional environment seems to have an important effect upon our health. We know that a bad temper can produce constriction of the bowels or produce an ulcer of the stomach through an excessive flow of digestive juices (namely hydrochloric acid).

None of these old people I met had any warlike tendencies or characteristics. They seemed to enjoy harmony and wanted to get along with people. They respected other people and wanted others to respect them. They seemed to cultivate a consciousness that radiated good will. Sick thoughts, destructive activity, malicious feelings all help to degenerate the body by sapping its vitality. These destructive impulses from the brain can cause a breakdown in the cellular structure throughout the body. Scientists believe we have our life span written in the DNA and RNA factors. It is here that we dete-

3

riorate or die, or have a long life and good health.

There is much to be said about factors that help postpone the aging processes of the body and aid in keeping the pattern of genetic information as clean as possible.

The DNA and RNA factors have been researched these last years and a great deal of work has been done by Dr. Benjamin S. Frank in his experimental work. Vitamin B, as in Brewers Yeast, is one of the richest foods in nucleic acids and while it does have all the elements of the Vitamin B complex it is not as complete a food because it does not contain all the minerals. Sardines (the smaller the better) are very high in nucleic acids because they are a whole food. I don't think that anything squirms faster and moves better in proportion to its size than the tiny sardines. Dr. Frank has found a definite effect in regard to the brain and nervous system and that there was an increase in mental acuity when using the RNA and DNA factors.

DIGESTION

The most recurrent problem of most people of advancing years is that of indigestion. The elderly people whom I met were living on those foods which were easiest to digest. They ate leaves and greens and such other foods that lower the blood pressure, which usually tends to become higher as people grow older. These elderly people were living on foods that needed less hydrochloric acid to digest, namely clabbered milk which is used so abundantly by the Roumanians, Turks, and Russians.Clabbered milk, which involves a process of curdling the milk, is essentially a pre-digested product requiring little if any hydrochloric acid in the digestive process. We are speaking, of course, of raw, unpasteurized milk when we say that it is one of the best foods to feed the brain and nervous system. This strictly is a whole food because of the uncooked process and one of the best foods to feed the brain and nervous system. The animal product itself carries a magnetism and a power; a force that can be used by the body and directly by the nervous system as it absorbs this magnetic quality. We find it in the animal products of milk, and many times eggs. All the old men I met seemed unusually free of all signs of congestion with its attendant diseases and problems. Their elimination channels were working at peak efficiency. These people answer nature's call immediately and cannot understand such a thing as constipation. They do not realize there is such a thing as skipping a day. They knew that they must drink plenty of liquids and that the odor of the urine is

4

controlled mainly by the amount of water one drinks. They drank plenty of water and perspired freely, keeping the skin as an eliminative organ in good activity. They tended to follow the digestive process relating to animals by having a bowel movement after every meal.

BOWELS

In my work covering 48 years of practice, and having had the privilege of working with some 100,000 patients, I came to the conclusion long ago that the prevention of disease is essential to the prolongation of life. Disease weakens the body. Continual coughs, colds, sinus disturbances, mastoid troubles, catarrhal discharges, in fact any bodily discharges tend to sap and devitalize the body. To prevent disease we must be aware of the importance of elimination. The old people I met in various parts of the world lived in a climate and at an altitude where their skins were active eliminative organs. However, their summers were never so hot that they lost excessive sodium salts through perspiration. Their higher altitudes forced these people to breathe more deeply. This helps the lungs to throw off toxic materials, catarrhal congestions, phlegm or mucus through the bronchial tubes. Their activities induced deeper breathing thus developing the oxygen centers of the brain. Climbing about on their rough terrain necessitated taking deep breaths which, of course, helped to develop an excellent and sturdy lung structure. They did not have dehydrated bodies resulting in a concentrated urine that is retained in the bladder.

This brings us to one of the common problems associated with elderly people. Much of the uric acid and the related joint troubles are caused, I am sure, by the retention of urine. This causes it to be reabsorbed by the body, and a good deal of it can settle in the joints. The genito-urinary tract is largely responsible for most prostate gland trouble. I am convinced that the health of the glandular system is dependent upon the perfect functioning of the genito-urinary system.

Of all the eliminative organs, the bowels are the most important. These old men I met always heeded nature's call. They seemed to have no inhibitions and availed themselves of all the surrounding countryside. They were never too busy and never waited 'til later. Modern civilization is very lax on this hygienic point. They think it's normal to have a bowel movement every other day or even longer. I've had patients who had bowel movements once in two weeks. I've even

5

known doctors who have thought this was not too serious a matter. Yet, when the bowels were taken care of and encouraged to function normally, many of the other symptoms which the patients may have had, such as menstrual disorders, lung congestions, runny ears, vanished. Elimination is of utmost importance. Toxic wastes must be expelled from the body regularly and efficiently.

The medical world has developed various antibiotics to combat bowel-related infections and diseases, such as their sulfa drugs. The use of these drugs, however, destroy the friendly bacteria of the bowels. This, in turn, inhibits natural digestive action; and so we find ourselves running around in the proverbial vicious circle. To have a healthy body, a normal acid-alkaline balance must be maintained in the intestinal tract. We must have at least an 80% balance of acidophilus bacteria as compared to the destructive 20% of bacillus coli or other degenerative bacteria. Modern civilization has made many improvements where sanitary conditions are concerned. We've cleaned our streets, disposed of garbage, and devised elaborate sewage systems. How ironic it is that we haven't learned to clean out our own bowels.

Young people are much too preoccupied to be concerned about preserving their youth—a mere fleeting period of 15 to 20 years, or so. Only after youth has fled, does its recapture preoccupy thought. We all need to learn as early as possible how to help our bodies function as normally and naturally as possible. These venerable old men did this without even being aware of it. We must learn to do this also. Because our environment may be quite different from theirs, we may have to exercise a conscious effort to approximate as closely as possible the principles followed by these long-lived individuals. Many are striving for money with all their might and main. We glorify these people thinking that success is what we would like to have. Many a man has ruined his life coming from the farm and going to the city to seek his fortune. We should be glorifying the youthful, the cheerful and the heart-warming things coming from a natural life. Age is not a matter of years, but of feeling. Youth is the power of feeling things freshly, greeting our next moment with life and energy. It is finding joy in the uncommon, being eager and enthusiastic. We have to refuse to count the cost. We cannot go through life counting our losses. These will take up too much of our time that is necessary for the youth of the future and we end up exhausted. Phillip James Bailey says we should live in deeds, not in years, in thoughts, not breaths, in feelings, not in figures on the dial. We should not count time by heart-throbs. He lives the most who thinks the most, feels the noblest, acts the best.

Most of us have heard of Bulgarian buttermilk and the Bulgaricus Acidophilus. This particular culture was named for this country because there is a greater proportion of people over 100 years of age there than anywhere else on earth. We can assume therefore that this Bulgarian acidophilus culture, this friendly bacilli of the bowel, must have something to do with this interesting statistic. The Bulgarians also set aside the left over whey from the clabbered milk for the elderly. By studying the chemistry of foods we know that whey is high in sodium and it is this sodium element which helps dissolve hardness in the body.

During my study at the Battle Creek Sanatarium, Dr. John Harvey Kellogg told me that there are four or five things that break down the friendly bacteria in our bowel more than anything else. They are meat, cooked food, chocolate and coffee. This was the reason why I stopped drinking coffee. We should do all we can to build up the friendly bacteria in our bowel, by limiting our intake of meat. In fact, if we really wanted to choose the better way, we would choose an almost entirely meatless diet. We could go still further by cutting out much of the cooked food we eat and putting raw foods in their place. We should definitely make it a practice to start out meals with a raw salad.

There are 1,800 tons of laxatives sold every year in the United States. There isn't a more lucrative business to be found anywhere. Laxatives irritate the liver causing a greater amount of bile to flow into the intestinal tract. Although the toxic waste accumulation may be taken care of for the time being, the bowel trouble is not corrected. When the liver isn't working properly, neither will the bowels work properly. When the liver and bowels are functioning as they should, there are no problems with hemorrhoids. Doctors usually have to consider the liver in their treatments. because sick people invariably also have liver problems. Every degenerative disease seems to involve the liver. When we have conditions that could metastasize from other problems in the body and go to the liver, it can be serious. The liver is the detoxifier of the body. For absolute cleanliness, we must have a clean liver. The bile must flow freely into the intestinal tract.

There is an interesting parallel to consider between two orders of the Catholic religion—the Trappist monks and the Benedictine monks. The Trappists are vegetarians and include Bulgarian buttermilk in their austere diet. The Benedictines, on the other hand, are heavy meat eaters and include many rich foods in their meals. As a group their cholesterol level is extremely high and the incidence of heart attack is likewise high. This is not the case with the Trappist monks.

Dr. Wilfred Shute, one of the leading authorities on Vitamin E, claims that it is a superb anti-thrombin. He claims it is excellent to dissolve clots and to prevent them from forming when taken internally. The elderly people I met on my travels seemed to have plenty of this in their diets with natural grains and seeds.

Dr. Roger J. Williams in his book "Nutrition Against Disease" says that the consumption of lecithin is a useful and preventive measure in disease and especially good for cholesterol. Cholesterol has been one of the factors to overcome in elderly people in this country and it is so rampant that many doctors are concerned about the increase because of our poor diet. Cholesterol deposits keep the blood from flowing freely through the arteries and especially from getting into the brain in the proper quantities. Fried foods are probably the greatest contributors to cholesterol forming in the body besides heated oils. This was one thing that was brought out by the elderly in the Hunza Valley. When I asked about their diet, they said, "Keep away from heated oils." How they knew this, I do not know.

I learned from these marvelous elderly people around the world that their diets followed the seasons. Although these people never heard of the word "diet", yet, in my opinion they were following a perfect diet. By eating fresh food and following the seasons, their bodies were getting all they needed. In each season we find that certain mineral elements predominate in certain vegetables and fruits. In the springtime, red strawberries are high in sodium. When blackberries come in, they are high in iron. The watermelon season makes silica available for our bodies. When nuts are abundant, we get the manganese we need for the memory and brain. Sesame seeds are high in lecithin, an important brain and nerve food. By eating the foods that are abundant in certain seasons, we acquire a reserve and are ready for the next season. Another thing we shouldn't overlook is our need for chlorophyll which is found in all the greens we eat. Besides being one of the best deodorizers for the body, it is also the best cleanser of the intestinal tract. You can learn more about this very important element in our book, "Health Magic Through Chlorophyll."

On my visits I realized the old people were not particularly aware that they have lived in the ideal climate, lived the ideal life mentally, lived at the proper altitude and all the other factors that go into the kind of life that brings fullness as well as longevity.

Their power to do the daily work in their gardens and fields was generated from a survival principle. It was inherited through their genes and gave them the will to continue, accomplish and motivate themselves to have plenty for tomorrow, living fearlessly with no past regrets or sorrows. They had something to look forward to that was worthwhile, happy and enjoyable. Above all, they were eating foods that were good for their bodies, and nourishing every cell and part of the body.

The important survival foods were all used and they are seeds, sprouts, berries and chlorophyll. They used the seeds of the sesame, sunflower and squash as well as others. Mung, lentil and many beans, grains and seeds were sprouted. They ate blackberries and cherries in season and dried the surplus for winter months. Chlorophyll was of course used as a green, but was eaten even with garlic. When they ate the bulb, they ate the leaves as well. They used whole foods. When they ate peas they used the pod. When they ate fruits they also used the pits. This will all be covered fully in our book "SURVIVE THIS DAY."

A short while ago a couple of men living in the jungles on islands off Japan were discovered. These men had survived for over 30 years on bugs, grasshoppers, ants, etc. They did not know the war was over but stayed there waiting until an officer came to tell them. But they *had* to survive until they got that message. I believe it is this survival quality in the elderly people who have lived so long that has kept them going day after day. They do not anticipate the disease and degeneration that most people expect.

It was Metchnikoff, the Russian bacteriologist, who said that senility is brought on by auto-intoxication, or through the absorption of toxic wastes in the large intestine. These poisons are taken back into the body thereby affecting and infecting all the organs of the body. Metchnikoff claimed that the harmful effect of this toxic material could be neutralized by changing the intestinal flora. By making a study of the intestinal vegetation, he found that certain types of sour milk had an anti-putrefactive property. He based his theories on the fact that fermentation develops in an alkaline environment. Consequently, because certain lactic acid bacteria develop in sour milk, the increase of other bacteria is retarded.

When fluids fail to carry off the excrements of the cell they degenerate, become senile and show signs of dying. Alexis Carrell kept the heart of a chicken alive for 30 years through the process of cleansing and proved Metchnikoff's findings that decrepitude and early death are due to poisons in the blood. "Purge the blood of its poisons," said Carrell, "and it (the blood) becomes a flowing fountain of youth."

Dr. Carrell also researched and proved that life lengthens if animals are fasted during certain fixed periods and that man's longevity could probably be augmented by similar procedures. He said that "fasting purifies and profoundly modifies or improves our tissues." The benefits of fasting are in accordance with our Key of Temperance. Scientific testing bears this out, also. Dr. Ross experimented with two groups of rats and found that by restricting the amount of food intake in one group they lived approximately 500 days longer than those who ate all they wanted.

The "American Journal of Clinical Nutrition," August, 1972, reported that a competent group of experts in the field agreed that the food intake, when restricted, even to the place where it might be considered an under-nourishing diet by the ordinary standards, lengthened the life and improved the health and even reduced the susceptibility to the diseases of the aged. Exton-Smith in the Journal observes that the diet that promotes the fastest growth brings a shortened life and hastens maturity. Fast growth is not desirable.

Another aspect of Temperance is illustrated by the life of Louis Conaro who lived over the age of 100 after he had been given up to die in his 40th year. At that time he had become quite dissipated from a very riotous life and resolved to reform. The first thing he did was to adopt strict rules of frugality for eating and drinking. He did gentle exercises. His book maintains that "one has to decrease intake of food in order to preserve health. Large quantities of food cannot be digested by old and feeble stomachs. By eating small amounts the stomach is not burdened and need not wait long to have an appetite . . . I eat only 12 oz. of solid food a day consisting chiefly of bread, broth, egg, mutton and perhaps chicken or pigeon and some kinds of fish such as pike, all of which are proper for old men." It was a sober and regular life that gave him his long years and he died without any pain in an alert frame of mind.

Galen, the physician who died in 270 A.D., aged 140, informs us that he always ate and drank sparingly irrespective of his appetite. Though of delicate constitution, he attributed his longevity to his temperance. Cardinal deSalis, archbishop of Seville, died in 1785 at the age of 125. He observed that he "led a sober, studious, but not a lazy or sedentary life." His diet was sparing.

WORRY

In discussing the mental side of life, we should realize that worry is the worst form of suicide. It is a slow form of self-destruction. Worry is the real cause of death in millions of cases. "One hour of worry is one hour in hell," writes James E. Dodds in his book "How To Master Worry."

Fear and worry are destructive to health, whereas happiness can be felt by every cell of the body. Man can also be motivated through the use of certain words and sounds that have a vibratory effect on the body. Using a fine vocabulary and speaking in kindly tones can have a most beneficial effect upon the cell structure of every organ in our body. We may wear ourselves our and burn ourselves out long before our time. Shirili Mislimov, 167 year old Russian, said that we cannot carry too much weight, for it is the thin horse that wins the race. We cannot be overly ambitious or competitive. Mislimov told researchers that he has always been satisfied with his role in life and that he has always practiced self-control. He told them that he rarely worries. In visiting these elderly people, we asked them about worrying and most of them seemed to have none or at least they said they didn't. Feeling youthful has nothing to do with one's chronological age. It is cheerfulness, enthusiasm, and eagerness. It is the cultivation of a fresh outlook.

GLANDS

The elderly people we met who had reached long lives were married. They were taking good care of each other and had the feeling of security. All the elderly men we met were sexually active even into the latter part of their years. Mr. Gasanov of Russia fathered his last child at 93 years of age.

Scientists such as Porter, Driel, Randvis noted that by feeding mice on foods devoid of Vitamin B (such as polished white rice) they witnessed a relatively early degeneration of the sexual glands. From a biological point of view their aging consisted mainly in supplanting the glandular tissue by connective tissue. This is identical to the process of old age. Through experiments with men it has been found that during famines, the spermatozoa disappear from the testicles. The ovaries of a starving female animal lose their ability to produce eggs. The sexual glands degenerate and die. This produces a complex problem in the body because we are "as young as our glands." The adrenal cortex is broken down through constant fear, problems and troubles and not giving this gland time to recuperate from constant activity. In time, this affects the sex gland, and in turn produces senility.

Diseases and climates have an effect on glands and they could become hypo-functional or hyper-functional accordingly. Higher altitudes quicken the thyroid gland, the lower the altitude, the lower the functioning or even a hypo-function of the thyroid. Constant illness or drainage of the body of life forces through coughing, colds, and debilitating disease will in time drain and weaken the endocrine glandular system where we will be tired, unable to accomplish and meet the new day as we should.

It is unusual to hear that you are in pretty good shape for your age. Most people expect diseases the older they get and you are supposed to "look your age." Osteoporosis is common among elderly for as we grow older we do not regenerate as well. Heart disease, atherosclerosis, hypertension, diabetes, arthritis and senile dementia are more common as we grow older; but it is necessary and possible to prevent them. Ten per cent of the American population is now over 65 and about 86% have one or more of the degenerative diseases. The older individuals have a maximum life span in the human genes programmed from their inheritance.

Leslie Orgel of the Salk Institute believes that almost any error—if it occurs in a critical enzyme—could result in a chain reaction of errors: an error catastrophe that could interfere with, or altogether stop protein manufacture. I believe that as one organ breaks down it interferes with the function of every other organ in the body and we need them all to be in good order for long life and good health.

Hormones are being used today to increase our life span and to bring us greater health. The female hormones protect the heart muscles in rats, and this may be one of the reasons that women have fewer heart attacks than men.

The prostate cells of old rats don't seem to synthesize RNA as well as when they were young. All the scientists and researchers today are beginning to recognize that it is the genes, the inherent quality of the person, that determines how the enzymes are carried out throughout all life and how the glands continue to function.

Many scientists are working on aging problems today; some are working on the glands, another on the liver, another with the heart, another with the pancreas. Then we come to specific factors and in trying to make up for some missing factors when the person is born by putting them back into the body, they are trying to release certain hormones through stimulation. They are even trying to find if there is such a thing as a death hormone in the body. This is brought out because a deficient hormone activity closely resembling aging is taking place. If a person was young enough the body could be changed. Dr. W. Donner Denckla of La Roche Institute of Molecular Biology in Nutley, New Jersey, believes that the clock of aging takes place in the brain.

William E. Gladstone, one of England's prime ministers, lived a long time. He was elected four times—at the ages of 59, 71, 77, and 83. He did a prodigious amount of work but he never seemed under pressure. No one ever remembers seeing him in a hurry. He lived simply and was extremely domestic in his taste. He was frugal without being abstemious. Plain living and high thinking were his standard. The popular story about him was that he attributed his good health and vigor to chewing his food 20 times before swallowing it. He ate very slowly and he made it a rule not to talk about business affairs or politics after he retired from his business in the evening. He also believed that physical exercise was very important. When he could not enter into outdoor sports, he spent his time chopping down useless trees.

A good example is Reverend Henry Grigs Weston who was President of Crozer Theological Seminary in Chester, Pa. He said, "When I was 30 years old, I broke down so that for two months I did not speak a loud word and everybody thought I was going to die. I didn't die, but the following summer I was not able to do any work and I had time to think how a man ought to live. I made up my mind, and formed my plans, which I have followed ever since, and I have done a great deal of work. I can't speak as to the quality of it, but the quantity has been all that I can ask.

The first necessity of life is air to the lungs, and so I began that summer the practice of filling my lungs every day for ½ an hour at a time with fresh air, the best I can find. That custom I have followed ever since, and every day now I see that my lungs are expanded to their full capacity with the best air obtainable.

The second principle I adopted was that the sun was the source of health. And I can look out from the room where I sleep at the sun shining.

The third principle is that God made night for sleeping. It is my duty to sleep when the night comes, and it is my duty to get up in the morning when the morning comes. And I dropped all my night work. I did not break these rules except by absolute necessity. When asked about his diet, he said, "I did not diet myself more than this. I am a small eater, have no love for high living, and do not eat rich foods. I had smoked and used tobacco for 8 years. I was an excessive smoker. When I got out of tobacco, often I would ride 10 miles to lay in a stock. I made up my mind that I would not be a slave to the habit and I quit."

He wrote these things in his 85th year. He keenly relished a walk from 1 to 3 miles daily.

Young men must do most of the world's strenuous work, but we still call on the elderly for final decisions, for experience and wisdom are needed to pursue a right course. The elderly should expect to continue utilizing their abilities. I believe we could do a great service to humanity by setting up educational groups for therapy, sharing experiences, and conselling people as they are gowing older. One group could begin at age 50, another at 60, 70 and beyond so people could learn more about each stage of life. As we transform and grow into different levels of activity we should know what our bodies are capable of doing; what to eat and how to adjust. It is interesting and refreshing to read how Goethe worked at his daily task even past the age of 80. Time did not seem to weaken his intellect or slacken his energy. Some of his most beautiful poems were written when he was about 75 years of age. With a little research one could turn up countless interesting accomplishments of people commonly considered to be past their prime. The very fact of attaining a ripe old age and manifest good health is in itself no small accomplishment.

In the life of Victor Hugo we see that some of his great works, such as "Les Miserables," was written when he had passed 57.

Humbolt illustrates what a man is worth intellectually after 60 or 70 years of age. He did many great things before that time, but after age 60, at the request of Emperor Nicholas of Russia, he undertook a scientific expedition to the North of Asia to explore the Ural and Altai Mountains, Chinese Dzungaria and the Caspian Sea. When he was 74 years of age he began to compose "Cosmos," essay of a physical description of the universe, which had been unanimously recognized as one of the greatest scientific works ever published. The fourth and last volume was not issued until 1858, one year before his death at the age of 90.

Anatomical experiments and investigations show that the chief characteristics of old age are deposits of earthy matter of a gelatinous and fibrous nature in the human system. A man is as old as his arteries; it is the degeneration and weakening of the arteries that shorten life. The largest item the body needs is oxygen. This gas is carried by the red blood corpuscles. Each is about 1/3200th of an inch in diameter. The blood contains from twenty-five to thirty trillion of them. Their total combined surface is almost an acre (an acre is approximately 44,000 square feet). We must be sure this blood is free of all toxic material. All body waste must pass off through the lungs, the bowel, the skin and the kidneys. The absorption of polluted air into the blood through the lungs causes rapid changes in the corpuscles in the body. The capillaries are found in these fine blood vessels of the lungs and lie in direct contact with the walls of the air sacs and are just big enough to allow the red corpuscles to pass through them in single file. The corpuscles carry the oxygen through these capillaries to the different organs in the body for developing heat and burning up the waste in the body and for developing good digestibility of our foods.

Thomas Parr, a native of Shropshire, England, died in 1635 aged 152. He married at the age of 88, seeming no older than many at 40. He was brought to London to see Charles I. He fed high, drank plentifully of wines by which his body was overcharged. His lungs were obstructed and the habit of his whole body quite disordered. In consequence, there could not be that speedy dissolution. If he had not changed his diet and habits he might have lived many years longer. When his body was opened by Dr. Harvey he was found to be in most perfect shape. The heart was thick, fibrous and fat. His cartilages were not even ossified as is the case in all old people and the only cause to which death could be attributed was a mere plethora brought on by luxurious living in London.

During moderate activity, all the blood in the body passes

through the lungs more than 100 times an hour. If the air we inhale is too warm the blood vessels in the lungs expand, and the corpuscles are unable to pick up the oxygen so readily, with the result that the person experiences a feeling of suffocation. One reason why cool air is so bracing is that it is more condensed and contains more oxygen. There is sometimes as much as 25% more oxygen in 0° air than in 100° above zero. In the direct ratio as the blood becomes stagnant, impure and abnormal, will all organs and parts of the body decline from health. This is not disease, but degeneration which portends a steady decline in health. Not time, but toxic products in the blood produce the senile changes we call old age. It is the body that makes blood and purifies it. Nothing else can do the work. Not even the greatest chemist can make a drop of blood. Our body has to do this. If we purge the blood if its poisons, the blood becomes a flowing fountain of youth.

Many scientists are working on aging problems today; some are working on the glands, others on the liver, others with the heart or pancreas. I hope with all the scientific work going on today, that the result isn't a mere stretching out of the years of senility. Their aim should be that the greater longevity will include good health and vigor. The architects of the body and the tissue builders are the live foods we eat. They have the natural embryo, the germ, the spark of life. To build this physical life properly, we must derive vitality from the food we eat. We won't find this vitality in sickly foods. It is when the body doesn't receive all the materials it requires to make a good body that we grow old and feeble. I am convinced that the soul and spirit never grow old, for the soul is as spritely and young in the 100-year-old person as in the 20-year-old. The elderly people I met could be said to be living in a "Garden of Eden." They did not have French cooks, drug stores or supermarkets. They did not have hospitals either with cola drink dispensers in the hallway for the patients.

Food is man's only truly reliable medicine and foods do cure, just the same as wrong foods and drinks may kill us. There are ten times as many scientists and nutritionists working in the field of animal health as in human health in the U.S., according to Dr. George M. Briggs of the University of California at Berkeley. He has said that the average American's diet is a national disaster. When our food is unnatural and devitalized, when it is polished, when it is only a part of what it should be, when it is impure from an accumulation of sprays, additives, etc., then this food is no longer life-giving and regenerative.

Octogenarians are invariably frugal eaters. Miguel Solis of Bogota, San Salvador, was at least 180 when at a Congress of Physicians, Dr. Luis Hernandez reported his visit to this locally famous man. "We are told that he only confesses his age to be 180 years, but his neighbors confirm that he is considerably older. One of the local citizens says when he was a child Solis was recognized as a centenarian." His signature in 1712 was discovered among those who assisted in the construction of a Franciscan convent in San Sebastian. Dr. Hernandez found this wonderful individual working in his garden and described his "skin to be like parchment; his hair as white as snow and covered his head like a turban." He attributed his long life to his careful habits; eating only once a day for a half an hour because he believed that more food that could be eaten in one-half hour could not be digested in 24 hours. He was accustomed to fast on the 1st and 15th of every month, drinking on those days as much water as possible. He chose the most nourishing foods and took no things cold." The LANCET, Sept. 1878.

★ ★ ★

The famous patriarch of the New England pulpit, Dr. Nathaniel Emmons, vigorous at 95, was heard to say, "I always get up from the table a little hungry."

★ ★ ★

The enormous physiological task of digesting and excreting daily pounds of food not actually needed is something the wise elderly people never impose upon themselves. Instead he expends his vitality in thought, in working, and in living out his century. We live not so much because of what we eat as because of what we do not eat. A Dr. George Cheyne says that the aged should lessen the quantity and lower the richness of their food gradually as they grow older, even before a manifest decay of appetite forces them to do so. There are many forms of indigestion and states of imperfect nutrition of the whole body that are caused by bolting down one's food.

Speaking of the conditions for longevity and man's usefulness in old age, Dr. Harvey Washington Wiley, Chief of the Government Bureau of Chemistry, said that to live long one must live moderately both as to eating and drinking. Age hardens the veins. Tissue is not built up as in youth. Starting with a strong, healthy body, and then living temperately is important. The next requisite is work. Idlers rust out. Recreation is also an essential part of the recipe for old age. Amusement is as necessary as sustained endeavor. One bit of advice that I would like to share with you regards the sealed book of 100 pages bearing the title, "The Onliest and Deepest Secrets of the Medical Art" which was found among the effects of the celebrated Dutch physician, Dr. Herman Boerhave, after his death in 1738. The book was sold at auction for $10,000 in gold. After the seal was broken the buyer had discovered that 99 pages were blank. Only the title page bore this inscription in the doctor's own hand, "Keep your head cool, your feet warm, and you'll make the best doctor poor."

Have you ever wondered just how long a man could live under perfect conditions? Some people theorize that the reason we do not attain a great age is that we don't have the proper energy and brain force. Others say that the chemical inactivity in and around each cell nucleus results in cellular starvation. Aging is one of life's biggest mysteries. Professor Chebotarev has said that the mountain centenarians eat really healthy food. It is all home-grown, it doesn't have chemical additives, and it is really healthy food. There is no frozen food in the Caucasus! In the Caucasus, according to Professor Chebotarev, 49 out of every 100,000 people live to the age of 100 years or longer, while in the United States there are only 3 out of every 100,000 that live over 100 years. After having practiced for nearly 50 years and with a great number of patients, I am convinced that a correct diet and the right physical build can keep a person well. This diet must be balanced. No matter what the age, there is a cause for declining health, beauty, youthfulness and vigor. An incorrect diet can produce illness, and our complexion and sprightliness can slowly fade. A low-iron diet leads to anemia and a low-calcium diet leads to exhaustion. We must watch our civilization more than anything else, for our modern foods are no longer foods. Man is trying to get a good body out of foodless food. John D. Rockefeller, as an old man, offered a million dollars to anyone who could help him digest a ham sandwich. No one was able to help him and no one ever could. We must learn that acidity is the grim reaper, taking the youth from our bodies. The food chemists, food scientists, food analysts, and the food manufacturers will be responsible for our health in the future. It is the canners, the millers and the cooks who are the ones we have to watch. They are the ones who can bring us to our grave at an early age. The foods we are getting today are leading us to the hospital, the operating table and the undertaker a lot earlier than necessary. It is in getting closer to nature, closer to the garden, and further from the drug store that we are going to have good health and salvation and a long life.

THE HILLS OF ESCONDIDO: A LONG-LIFE CENTER

I believe that Escondido could have the name of probably one of the best of our long-life centers in the whole country. The reason I say that is this: we have hills here that compare to the hills of those people who have lived a long life, hills that range from 2,000 to 5,000 feet. And if you should look about here for yourself, you would see that we are halfway between the desert and the ocean. You would not drink stagnant water here. Also, the finest thing you can live in is air that is in motion. If you were to consider it, the hot desert air pulls that cold air from the ocean into the desert and right over this place. If you watch the clouds, they are in motion. And when you are around here, the air is in constant motion. There is no stagnant or humid air here.

It is not just a happenstance that the largest telescope in the world is located at Mt. Palomar, only 25 miles from Escondido. The lens is a 200" lens, and by having it at this altitude they claim to have the clearest air anywhere in this area. The engineers, in setting up the telescope, say this is the finest place for the observation of heavenly bodies anywhere in California or in the southern part of the United States.

This latitude is exactly the same as the latitude where one can find the elderly people. They enjoy the same kind of soil, the same kind of growth of fruits and vegetables; and they had a lot of Keys in this type of climate to keep them well and living the long life.

Escondido is on the same latitude as Greece; Alexander the Great's birthplace was in Macedonia. He was one of the strongest men to begin with, and considered strength one of the necessary factors a person needs in order to conquer. Greece, the upper part of Italy, Turkey, Iraq, Iran, the southern part of Russia, etc., are all found in this same latitude; and I consider it to be a belt where people can live this long life and have the greatest strength. That is why I think Escondido could be a wonderful center for long life and good health.

In the Escondido area we have grapes growing beautifully. Unfortunately, many of the vineyards are being removed as more commercially profitable ventures come into the area. And when you stop and think about it, all the elderly men lived where grapes grow. Escondido was known as the grape country here in California at one time. In fact, we have a park right in the middle of Escondido called the grape park. And in the buggy days, people used to come up from San Diego to have their conventions and their meetings during the grape season in the grape park here in Escondido.

You will find that where all of these long-life people live, there are the same climatic conditions and mountain conditions existing close to Escondido. It is not just a happenstance that Alpine, California, has been investigated by the government; and it was found that there is more sunshine in this community than in other places around southern California. This is a place where they live around 3,000 feet, and they have the finest of sunshine possible.

It is not just a happenstance that the government has been investigating Fallbrook as probably the finest place for good air in this area, and has checked to find that these people have less pollution in the air than in any other surrounding community. The air has been found to be the clearest and the purest in Vista, Fallbrook and Escondido of any places that the government has tested. The government tests have also tried to determine if children, living in this kind of air, have any trouble in tardiness, in attendance, and in the amount of colds and flu they have. The government is making these tests now in the schools to see if there is a difference between the rural schools and the city schools.

There are a number of other reasons why this particular area is good. First of all, you don't find any industrialization here in Escondido. They have kept out factories and the smoke they would subsequently produce. You find that the people live where there are a lot of avocados, and this tells us that this is a sub-tropical area. We find out that where the old men live there is always a lot of fighting going on. In one place in Russia, for instance, there have been over 200 wars fought in the last 2,000 years. And we found it is because they all wanted that particular part of that country. Who wouldn't want the country that can grow all the fruits, all the vegetables, all the varieties of foods from avocados to walnuts and almonds? In that kind of place, you would have everything you could possibly want or need.

In Escondido, there is a growing season of 12 months a year. You can't say that about New York. In fact, you can't say that about many parts of the country. And that is why I say that Escondido could be the place where we could have many centenarians living if people would just practice the fine art of dieting, exercising, probably a little jogging, and getting enough of the wonderful sunshine and pure air we have so much of here. There are many lovely things that we have in Escondido in order to lead a good life.

Chapter 2

Foods For Health

The first bottle of soda pop is not going to harm us; the first cigarette isn't going to produce a cancer. It isn't the first eating of any one food that produces a disease any more than the first drop of water will wear away that proverbial stone. It is the continuation thereof. Too much fried food, too many dumplings, condiments or processed foods wear away the good in our bodies.

Most of us already know that overeating may kill us, but how many of us know that many hot foods are dangerous in ANY quantity. To follow a meal with ice cream is wrong for many reasons. The cold is a shock to the system. Besides, most diners eat until they are already full before stuffing themselves with a dessert. Come to think of it, eating dessert is just a habit. Of course, we like it; sweets taste good, but there is such a thing as overdoing it. Cold desserts, especially, tend to contract the walls of the stomach and prevent the digestive juices from functioning properly.

If we would but realize these so-called minor things have their place in the economy of the body, we would eat with more wisdom. We would search more diligently for foods that will maintain health. We would make a tea from apple peelings that would probably do more for the kidneys than anything else; for that matter, it is constructive for ANY organ in our body that is broken down.

The skins of other fruits, besides the apple, as well as the skins of certain vegetables have valuable properties to affect different parts of our bodies. They should be in tonics and liquefied drinks. In every glass of carrot juice there are fifteen thousand units of Vitamin A.

Turnip juice contains the greatest catarrhal eliminator we have. Every asthmatic and bronchially-affected person should know the value of turnips. My experience alone in using turnips to build health would prove it one of the finest foods. I will not say it is the greatest, but I will say that with turnips alone you can do more for bronchial ailments, more for lowering the blood pressure, and more for getting Vitamin A into the body, than with any other food I know.

Soon after World War II, I met two soldiers, just discharged, who had spent four years in a German concentration camp. This pair lived on turnips and nothing else for the entire four years they were in prison. You will find it hard to believe, but they were both in perfect health. I might add that I never found cancer in any person confined in concentration camps during the war. That is because, when they did get food, it was simple food—not very good to taste, true, but not detrimental either.

The effects of a steady turnip diet among war prisoners is extraordinary. In many cases, they had better teeth when released than when captured. Of course, they were thin; turnips do not build fat on the body. Many of them had better complexions and better fingernails and hair. Their bodies were so influenced by the chemical elements in turnips that they had regular bowel movements. I have prescribed turnips for a good many people. I grow turnips on my Hidden Valley Health Ranch; white turnips that have the purple tops. Turnip greens were one of the nine greens we used in treating the little girl whose legs had been covered with ulcers for three years. The combination of greens healed them in three weeks.

One of our patients at the ranch suffered from asthma, catarrhal trouble and a 240 blood pressure. We put him on a thirty-day diet of nothing but turnips. We gave him turnip greens, turnip juice, raw and cooked turnips. Nothing but turnips for one month. When taken off the diet, he no longer had asthma or catarrhal trouble; his blood pressure was normal and he was down to his normal weight by losing 40 pounds. He was a picture of health. Compare this with the pills and potions he had been taking for years.

Dr. Quida Davis Abbott, head of the Department of Home Economics at the University of Florida, touched on this subject of diet in an address she gave before the National Dietary Food Association in Chicago.

Dr. Abbott stated: "Many Americans are mal-nourished. America is the richest nation in the world. Americans spend approximately 15 billion dollars a year on food, but reports from draft boards, physician's records and nutritional surveys indicate that a large segment of the population is misfed and underfed. The cause is simple; Americans do not eat enough of the right kinds of foods. One family in ten has a good diet, less than four in 10 have passable diets and more than 50 percent have poor diets. The lack of a proper nutritional education program in grammar, high school and college is one of the contributing causes to this dilemma.

"No nation can afford to have a large segment of its population among the underfed and misfed. Not only must we produce more food, but more people must know how to select a good diet and be willing to eat what they should."

A lack of calcium can cause cannibalism in animals. We have a lot of people today who are killing without any sense or logic behind it, and I believe that wars are caused from poor chemicalization and poor mineralization in people. If quarrels can be handled by remineralization, it is something for us to consider at the peace table. The size of the rat, his intelligence, can be controlled through feeding. Irritability and emotions can result from a mineral imbalance. Plants, when fed properly in the soil, need less spray, less injection. The same thing exists in man. He will need less injections, less dope to live on if he gets the proper food grown from the proper soil.

The soft body is the young body, the body filled with a lot of sodium. The hard body is what we call stiff and old. It is possible to be young at eighty or old at twenty. When we look back many generations we see that we had a different soil and a different climate from what we have today. It probably grew a better vegetation, larger and coarser, and man and the animals that lived off that vegetation were larger.

Typical Co-eds Live on Diet That Kills Rats

Ft. Collins, Colorado, Nov. 23— A "typical" co-eds diet would not keep a rat alive. A menu of chocolate cake, candy, pickles and soft drinks, declared by students and teachers in the nutrition laboratory of Colorado State College to be "just about typical" of what the college girl of today exists on, is slowly killing several white rats.

The food has been ground together, dried and fed to the rats for three weeks by 25 girls taking the nutrition course in the home economics division of the college. For three weeks the rats have gained only a few ounces, have lost most of their hair, have turned yellow and in general definitely show that they are on the way toward death from lack of proper food.

Cultured Products

I believe that if you cannot get a sweet raw milk, warm right from the animal—preferably a goat—you are better off to let the milk clabber. A lot of people wonder just what the proper way to clabber milk is. You cannot clabber pasteurized milk. We have to have raw milk. Put raw milk behind a stove or in a nice warm place. In a day and a half or so it clabbers. But put pasteurized milk behind a stove and it rots in a day and a half. You can't clabber pasteurized milk unless you start heating it and use fixatives. Now, the natural clabber is the best. On the other hand, you can use natural "fixatives". One of the nice ways to clabber milk is to use lemon juice; another one is to use apple juice. Then you can get lactic acid in the health food stores. This is one of the finest ways to clabber milk.

The Roumanian culture and the Bulgarian culture are responsible for a type of clabbered product we know as yogurt. There are all kinds of cultures that you can bring from one milk to another to clabber it. It is believed that milk clabbered by means of the Bulgarian culture is conducive to long life. Bulgaria has more people over a hundred years of age than any other country in the world, and yogurt is a staple in their national diet.

Almost every country has its variety of clabbered milk. You can go to Turkey where they have koumis; Indians use dahi; the Far East, "saya". It is a thing that we neglect in this country. However, we are getting acquainted with yogurt at last. In Switzerland when they go down to the "dairy" they call it a "yogurt store". Yogurt is a wonderful food, a wonderful bowel regulator. If you want to help get rid of gas and build up the body, take yogurt. Put a tablespoon of apple concentrate in it. This makes it the most wonderful bowel regulator that I know of. But probably you can't take it for one week and say that the bowels are any better—you've got to take it every day for

24

two months. Then you'll notice an improvement. This job takes a matter of months.

Elixir of Youth, Beauty
May Be Contained in Diet

Washington, Dec. 16 (NANA)— Diet, rather than some witch's brew or quack's nostrum, may be the long-sought elixir of youth and beauty.

There is accumulating evidence to this effect, says Dr. Hazel K. Stiebeling, director of the U.S. Department of Agriculture's Institute of Home Economics.

The thesis, she admits, is very difficult to prove because experiments are confined to short-lived animals. She outlines some of the evidence as it affects humans:

"From long experience with domestic and laboratory animals, Prof. Elmer V. McCollum of the University of Wisconsin and Johns Hopkins has concluded that human diets could contribute to what he called the 'preservation of the characteristics of youth' if they were richer than average in certain components of food—the nutrients calcium and Vitamins A and C. Outstanding for these nutrients are milk, dark-green and deep-yellow fruit, and vegetables and citrus and some other fruits.

Diet Prolongs Animal Life

Cornell University Experiments
With Controlled Feeding

Ithaca (N.Y.) April 2 (AP)— The day when a controlled diet may be utilized to increase, and possibly double, the production spans of life for cows, chickens, horses and other farm animals appears within reach today, on the basis of animal nutrition experiments at Cornell University.

Dr. C. M. McCay, of the animal nutrition department, said a three-year objective study in retarding the aging process and extending the productive life by limiting calories of the diet during the period of growth had revealed a technique by which animals can be kept "young" or allowed to proceed into senescence.

In laboratory experiments, Dr. McCay was able to double the normal life span of white rats by withholding food of high caloric content, such as sugars, from their diet. One group of animals fed an adequate diet with calories died after the normal life span of about 600 days.

Other groups lived on diets adequate in every respect excepting calories. The calories were added to the diet of one group when 300 days old, others at 500, 750 and 1000 days. Adding calories hastened the rodents to maturity, old age and death.

The group that did not have calories until 1000 days old survived all of the original 106 rats and lived more than 1200 days.

The average productive life of a dairy cow is computed at five years, a horse fifteen years and chickens from two and one-half to three years.

Dr. McCay said the experiment provided evidence that the rate of attaining maturity was an important factor in predetermining the total life span.

"This challenges," he observed, "the common concept that rapid growth develops the best bodies for long life."

The study showed, Dr. McCay said, that the powers of growth can be retained within the body of a rat for a period beyond the normal span of life, that the life span is flexible and that the extent to which it can be increased is an unknown value.

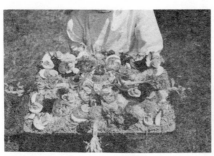

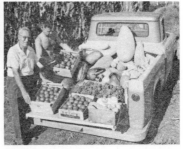

LIFE-BUILDING, YOUTH AND BEAUTY DIET

Life foods are fresh, living, thriving foods, direct from Nature's trees, bushes, gardens, plants and soil.

Foods containing the principle of life are:

Edible buds
Fruit blossoms
Alfalfa buds
Clover buds
Hop buds
Growing greens
Ripe fruit
Ripe berries
Nasturtium
Parsley
Celery hearts
Romaine lettuce
Leaf lettuce
Cabbage sprouts
Fresh tomatoes
Wilted spinach
Raw tender carrots
Collard
Shad roe
Blueberries
Blackberries
Wild cherries
Sprouts
Goat cream
Goat milk
Raw fresh milk
Chard
Raw egg yolks
Guavas
Mandarines
Raw nuts
Peppermint
Celery
Winter lettuce
Cos lettuce
Lamb's lettuce
Green onions
Raw spinach
Garlic
Papaw
Pecans
Fresh apples
Fresh asparagus shoots

Cucumbers
Roe
Genuine honey
Elderberries
Barberries
Bilberries
Fresh buttermilk
Goat butter
Cottage cheese
Curly cabbage
Chayote
Fresh blackcaps
Raw egg white
Fresh leeks
Mangoes
Grapes
Grape concentrate
Nettle salad
Papaya
Fresh pineapple
Fresh plums
Tender radishes
Wild strawberries
Swiss chard
Oranges
Goat milk whey
Fresh dates
Apple concentrate
Fresh pears
Tamarinds
Avocado
Chervil
Chinese cabbage
Marjoram
Yeast
Sundried figs
Loquats
Endive
Green peppers
Yellow tomatoes
Raw okra
Cole slaw

German prunes
Fresh fruit juices
Raisins
Muskmelon
Salad greens
Fresh peaches
Fresh raspberries
Fresh prunes
Strawberries
Sugar beet leaves
Sprouts that bloom
Black huckleberries
Tangerines
Watercress
Roquefort cheese
Olives
Sundried apples
Persimmons
Thyme
Chives
Edible greens
Mulberries
Fresh figs
Cowberries
Kumquats
Zante currants
Shallot
Turnip leaves
Caraway seed
Gherkins
Sapotes
Fruit sauce
Casaba
Adriatic figs
Mint
Bananas
Nectarines
Life tonics
Codliver oil
Vegetable broth
Fresh currants

BE SURE TO GET ALL YOUR HEALTH-BUILDING AND LIFE-GIVING FOODS FROM YOUR HEALTH FOOD STORE.

Chapter 3

Calcium and Inheritance

Dealing with man in general, and looking at him specifically with regard to what types these elderly men and women are, we find that they are predominantly calcium types of people. Each type of person expresses himself differently, works differently, looks and acts differently.

In the elderly people, you could see that they were bony, and that they had attracted calcium into their bodies, joints, bones, etc. Certain mental faculties put them in a classification of their own. The calcium man is a man of strength and purpose and of bone. He has a strong mental constitution, and this predominates throughout his body to influence his every thought, feeling, movement and action.

You can see that there is a similarity between the nature of the calcium element and the character of the man. He has metal in his blood and bones. He gravitates towards the mineral kingdom. He works with the earth and likes it; he is a stone-cutter, a quarry man, a coal miner, and he works in all kinds of solid materials. He doesn't care for soft fabrics and sentimental novels, poetry, music, etc. He is a stone man, so to speak; and you see this expressed so much in the work of the Hunza people in particular. The whole valley is stone. Their mountains come right down to them in almost solid stone. Their flumes are made with rock and stone. The roads on the side of the mountains are piled up with stone. They are builders and they work with their hands. They believe in work and in effort. They even make work out of play.

The calcium man is homely; and as a rule, he's very slow. He is earnest and persistent, very sturdy, determined and grim. He demonstrates his strength in times of opposition or when obstacles are put in his path.

This type can be slow and latent. They act slowly and

deliberately. He is like a winter apple; he develops slowly. Teachers think that he is short-witted or feeble-minded; for it is difficult for him to learn from books. He would rather blast rocks than memorize the Ten Commandments. He is like marble, slow to take impression. When, however, he has mastered a lesson, he can use it and hand it out with sledge hammer blows—with fists and hard work. He cares more for work, mud and action than he cares for school life.

We have these same types expressed in nature and in animal life. For instance, the ox is a calcium animal, while the cat, tiger and panther are sodium animals—quick in thought and quick in movement. The ox is bony and slow; the cat is quick. The ox is patient and domestic; the panther is wild and restless.

The calcium man has thick, hard and heavy bones. There are large and slow-acting brain cells within this person. They are slow in their nerve actions within the body. They seem to have a great love of truth and principles. In their activities they have a great inherent and physical power to study and to understand heavy-acting forces, including the mechanical forces. They want to be right in their judgment and they are quite exact in what they try to do.

When we put all of these mental and physical characteristics together, we have a physical momentum that is slow and regulated in its activity and speed. This is why these people live a long life. The calcium type is similar to a large driving wheel in a power house; he is slow and difficult to start, but he is also equally difficult to stop when once in motion. He carries right on by his own habits. Calcium is a hardy element, slow in motion. This is the reason that the calcium man is slow but sure. He makes every move count. He is one who uses a lot of reason, judgment, truth and accuracy. This is what makes him a good counsellor, and most of the members of the community seek him for advice.

Because of his build and his inherent characteristics, his mind, thought, body, speech and movements are slow acting. He doesn't wear himself out like the mental person whom we find in the United States today. The calcium type is slow to start, but slow to stop. They are slow to fall in love, but also slow to fall out of love. These people do not marry early in life, but believe in the married life and stay together until one of them dies.

Being slow in purpose, the calcium man keeps on coming, is slow to learn lessons, but is able to use them well. He is a hard master and a stern father, but a true lover and a good husband. Because the calcium man is slow and works by his own reason and is mostly his own teacher, you will find that he can be quite materialistic in his outlook. Many times he believes only in matter or concrete objects. He subjects everything to the court of reason. He is not too interested in the subjective world, or the spiritual world.

Living without sentiment, as he does, it is difficult for him to know too much about the aesthetic values of the world. He has to do things as he sees them done every day through habit, through the soil, and through the earth. Therefore, he has the same problem that science and theology have today—they haven't really come together and married well.

Because of the heavy amount of calcium in their bodies, we find that this type has good teeth and can keep them all of their life. They are set in their ways. These people usually select more milk, and their dishes are made mostly from cheese, cottage cheese, sour milk and buttermilk. They use coarse bread—their foods represent their type, and they develop their type from their foods. Their foods are rich in mineral salts that give them the well-balanced mineral bodies that they need for a long life and continued good health. You will find that they have a fondness for the calcium foods.

Calcium can bring good life, but can also bring on ossification if it isn't well balanced with other natural foods. However, these people living close to nature are able to balance their foods better than most calcium types that are born in civilization and live on "citified" foods. Because of their types of foods you will find these people are rich in the blood salts; and they have the capacity to metabolize and to retain these blood salts in abundance. These calcium men are seldom anemic; in fact, Mr. Gasanov's blood count was 6,500,000 when I met him at the age of 153.

Calcium people are great workers, almost reckless in their habits to get a good day's work done; but the bone metabolism requires great quantities of sodium salts in order to keep calcium in solution, or else it results in lime hardening in the body. All the elderly people were given whey from the cheese as a special drink for them; sodium is found highest in this whey extracted from the cheese. Therefore, these people had a lot of sodium salts to balance the calcium in the body and to keep their joints active and young, pliable and limber. They also got sodium in good quantities from all the sunshine fruits and vegetables. When we have a lack of sodium and fluorine salts in the body, it can lead to pneumonia and lung disturbances. One of the old men I visited had pneumonia at 114 years of age, but is still alive today at age 142. That was Mr. Toledo of Vilcabamba, Equador.

Mr. Gasanov of Russia had pneumonia when he was 148 years of age, and I met him at 153; so you can see that these people did get well. But the only problem they ever had anyway, was lung trouble or pneumonia, which possibly could come from the fact that they did not have enough of the sodium salts to balance the heavy chemical calcium that was taken into their bodies.

The calcium man is prudent in diet and habits. He is temperate and frugal in his eating habits, (temperance being the greatest Key of all), and never eats more than just what he should take. He is a slow eater, masticates well, chews slowly. This is why he is healthy and long-lived, more so than any other type of person. These calcium people usually have large families. They are sturdy men and women and can recuperate well from having children. They are the kind who can sleep in the cold, rain, storm and wind, and still recuperate well because of the heavy calcium salts in their bodies.

They are productive, vigorous and well-sexed unless they have abused their sexual system by excessive use of tobacco, whiskey, loss of sleep and habits that are detrimental to their health and vigor. Their habits are of the best to give them a well-balanced body, both glandular and health-wise.

Because of the religious principles laid down for the Hunza peoples, they have had no venereal diseases and germ life affecting their sex life until fairly recently. The Mir, himself, mentioned that it is only with civilization and people going to war in the lowlands, bringing back into the valley the impurities and germ life of bad sexual habits, that has caused the health and life span of these people to be cut down.

The endurance of these people is found mainly because of the bones. The red corpuscles of the blood are manufactured in the bone marrow. The number and vigor of these red corpuscles constitutes the vitality of the man. The calcium man has belief and faith in nature and in the laws of nature through his reason. His trust in people is weak, however; he will stick with a person only when he finds out and it has been proven to himself that the person is honest, reliable and trust-worthy.

The calcium man has more brain and bone to the square inch than any other type. He is compact, solid like cast iron, and can withstand heavy work. Calcium is the enduring element, and these are the men who really live a long life. They are built like oak; they can handle heavy strain. They have found that bone is almost as strong as cast iron, and nearly twice as strong as oak. The bones are enduring; calcium is an enduring element. The calciferous man is also enduring, strong and efficient, though slow to ripen.

Calcium people are ones that draw to them a great deal of calcium and phosphorus for bone building, and of course, they get it best out of a vegetarian diet. So many of the calcium people, and the long-lived people have been vegetarians or lean more towards the vegetarian foods. These foods when mixed with the dairy products which are high in calcium, helps to give them a more balanced diet.

The Hunzas live on a lot of fruit also, and these are high in sodium. Fruits are matured and sweetened by the sun which gives them their quality of a high sodium content, and this keeps the calcium in solution well, and does not allow arteriosclerosis, hardening of the arteries and hardened joints to form. This also is a good thing to balance out and keep in solution the heavy calcium found in dairy products, thus preventing the body from hardening too much.

Some people are very porous in bone structure and become very brittle. Calcium is found to be lacking in most people, but we find that the calcium man is different from most people because he draws the calcium to himself. It is found very heavily in his bone structure, which also gives him the long-life principles.

The sun is probably the calcium man's best friend, and all of the elderly men we have met have lived in a part of the world and in a country where grapes are found. An abundance of sunshine is the reason for all the fruits and vegetables in the particular area where they live. They live in the sun belts where it is not too hot, and where they derive the greatest value from the sun in the rarefied air where the sun is the clearest. The sun controls the calcium in our bodies because of the ultraviolet rays.

The average person, especially when he lives in the city, develops great nervousness and sensitiveness; there is an agitation of the nerves, mind and functions. But we find that the elderly people I visited do not have this problem. When they have enough calcium, they have complete control of the nerves. They have repose and they are resigned to the life around them. They are tranquil and they have the ability to fit in with their surroundings and environment without commotion or emotion.

Calcium combines well with silicon, magnesium, phosphorus and fluorine in the construction of bones and teeth. Calcium fluoride gives us the hardness needed in the teeth and the bones, and is a long-life element. We find that in drawing that extra calcium to their bodies, they also bring in fluorine when it is taken in their foods. By the way, fluorine is found only in raw foods, and is found highest in raw milk.

These elderly people I have met have very good digestion, and calcium always favor and assists the digestive ferments. In the laboratory we learn how calcium salts affect the ferment. Rennet is a ferment which is used in cheese-making to develop the curd of the cheese or milk. It is necessary, however, that the calcium contained in milk be perfectly soluble in order to curdle the milk. The cheese maker sometimes adds hydrochloric acid to the milk in order to increase the solubility of calcium salts. If calcium salts contained in the milk are taken out, the curds will never become thick. These people curdle the milk before eating it. In this way the digestive enzymes do not have to be taxed to the extreme, and the calcium is in a more soluble form. They never boil their milk, and the clabber milk is just kept at room temperature. Boiling the milk would also alter the calcium in the milk. This is another reason why they are able to live a long life, because they prepare their milk products properly.

If the calcium salts in the milk should be disturbed by whatever cause, whether by boiling the milk or otherwise, the rennet does not act properly upon the milk for cheese-making purposes. This is only brought out to show you the relationship of digestion with preparing the cheese and dairy products, and what the elderly people are using.

A lot of calcium salts in the blood prevent hemorrhages and help in the coagulation of the blood in case of any wounds. So, in the menu of the elderly people, it wasn't mentioned that calcium was necessary for a long life; but they were just eating the right things to continue and produce a long span of life, anyway.

When the calcium salts are diminished in our blood, vitality soon sinks, malnutrition takes place and soon the person can suffer from many different diseases. The teeth are fed from the inside. Calcium, fluorine, silica and other salts must be supplied or our dental work is increased. Tooth washes and pastes will do little good if we do not feed our teeth with the needed chemical elements.

If calcium salts are not supplied in normal quantities, we find that various processes of the body cannot be carried on in a healthy manner. With a deficiency of calcium salts the body will actually tear down its own structures in order to obtain the necessary calcium needed in vital tissues and bone metabolism, and in the internal secretions.

When the calcium supply is exhausted in the blood and in the secretions, the body goes to the only other available calcium source of supply—the teeth and the bones. When the calcium salts are extracted from a tooth, the understructure of the enamel is being undermined; and soon the thin enamel cracks or breaks, and putrifactive bacteria do the rest.

Even the fruit acids have a detrimental effect on the teeth. Sugar does not act upon the teeth directly but works upon them indirectly from the acids that it produces in the body. Calcium and sugar have an affinity for each other. If a person eats all sorts of sweet foods or glucose preparations that do not contain a sufficient quantity of calcium salts, these sugar or glucose preparations are likely to consume generous quantities of soluble calcium salts in the tissue and thus lessen the calcium in the system or in the tissues.

The more sugar there is in the system, the less calcium salts there will be. This is the reason why people should not eat so much sugar. It should also be noted that there are no sugar factories where these elderly people live.

Poultry farmers and egg producers know the value of

calcium for their poultry and for egg production. They go to the butcher for ground bones to feed to the chickens. They even feed their poultry cracked oyster shells, or some kind of food rich in calcium salts. In Petaluma, California they gave turnip greens to their chickens. Green kale was another favorite food for the chickens, and this is one of the highest foods there is in calcium and phosphorus. By feeding hens a diet rich in calcium, they will lay better and more eggs and have harder shells.

We must also remember that calcium is one of the chemicals that helps to build the cerebellum in the brain. The cerebellum has to be fed with good blood and plenty of it. The cerebellum superintends and makes many of the life functions more important, such as the synovial fluid for the joints. It has much to do with the thyroid gland, vocal cords, diaphragm, the heart muscle and the ventricles of the heart, sexual systems, many of the secretory glands, the knees, the small of the back and the hair. It also has control over the muscular coordination and locomotion. You see this working so well in these elderly people.

It influences the manufacture of the red blood corpuscles of the blood and the circulation, indirectly. When the cerebellum sinks, we grow old at any age—no matter whether the person is rich or poor, light or dark. Feeding the cerebellum helps to ward off old age.

This calcium characteristic in these people is inborn and carried down through the ages; it is hereditary. This quality was working in the parents long before the child was born.

An altitude of 4,000 to 10,000 feet with an abundant amount of ozone and with a warm, dry breezy climate is best for this type of person. They fare best in this altitude and climate. Exercise for this type of person should include working in the garden or fields. It should be almost vigorous, such as riding in wagons on rough roads, climbing hills, galloping on horseback, (exercises such as you find in the polo games of the Hunzas and in the back country activity of the Russians and Turks), and going back and forth on horseback. They have to have exercises that reach the bones and the joints and act upon the liver. To keep them in good health and living a long life, they have to have sunlight and outdoor work in their old age. This type of person is an early riser and goes to bed early.

They need a little bit more sleep than the average person, and it seems like they get it.

One of the great things we recognize is that these people who have a lot of calcium in their bodies have to take proper care of the stomach. This is one of the most important organs to take care of, and they do this with the clabbered milk. This gives them a food that is pre-digested and they don't need an excess amount of hydrochloric acid to curdle the milk, because they give their bodies pre-digested milk.

This type of person gets sick by degrees and also is cured by degrees. It takes sometimes 20 years of misuse and abuse to weaken or break down one of the vigorous organs in their bodies, and it may also take many years to cure them. But these people do not break down easily, because their environment is so pleasing and right for them that they are able to live a good, flowing life, so that they can be curing and preventing disease while they are living this long life.

The calcium man is born for health. These people have the strongest constitution, and they are so strong in bone that they are almost immortal! The most enduring man is the one with a lot of calcium in his body. If he would take good care of himself during his entire life, it is difficult to know when he would die. By having a lot of calcium in the body one has a tendency towards feats of strength, victory in wrestling, gallant deeds, equestrian sports, hunting, etc.

Calcium types disregard the demands of society or refined customs. They prefer common apparel, and are satisfied with working clothes. They defy customs, society and fashion. They have a working desire because they are capable; and working with the earth and with hard materials does not break down their bodies very easily. Because of their rugged frame, they have a natural inclination to till the soil. They have a preference for the simple mode of life and can be found close to nature in the forest, meadows, trees, etc.

When calcium is working in a strong, health body, the sexual system will also be strong. These people believe more in deeds than in faith. Calcium does not naturally allow for delicacy, tenderness or weakness. They do not travel much. They usually stay at home. It is their heredity and calcium phosphate that makes them what they are.

The people who live this long life can give a great deal of credit to their ancestors and environment. It is the natural calcium that they have inherited over a period of centuries that gives them this great strength and endurance. All the World Keys and principles that have helped them to live this long life have come to them unaware. They don't realize that the altitude, climate, foods, civilization and attitudes all have an effect upon us. They have the bodies to live these long lives and are just doing what comes naturally in their environment. Their endowment of calcium, in proper balance, is a main factor to living the long life in the best of health.

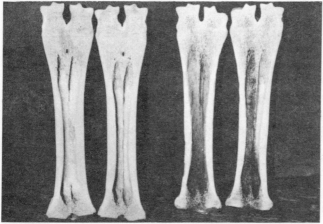

Bones are dependent upon calcium and phosphorus. They house the bone-making organ called bone marrow. The calcium types have the best bones and the best bone marrow tracts. This is where long life begins.

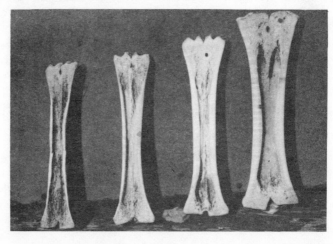

Chapter 4

Civilization

CIVILIZED MAN

Civilization has come upon us and has brought a lot of problems along with it, and one of the greatest of all problems, I believe, is man's using his mind in a more constructive way. It seems that we are cutting down on time, cutting down on distance, space seems to be becoming no object to overcome; but yet again, we find disease is increasing and many hardships from a humanitarian standpoint are on us. Our jails are full, our rest homes are overcrowded, billions of dollars are being spent in building new hospitals in the next few months. Certainly this is not a civilization that is looking toward preventing diseases and bringing the best of all to mankind's comfort, health and security.

However, I do believe we are going through an extreme transition period that will surely bend us to our knees with a desire for a better day for our families, for our children, for our living, for the foods that are served, for our financial system, and for our governing bodies. It is a crime that we have to fight in order to have good health when so much of an abundant life surrounds us. Day after day we hear reports about DDT being so harmful to the human body. We hear about crates of lettuce picked up by our government agencies because the lettuce has been sprayed too much and would be detrimental to the human body. Yet we do nothing to teach those who don't know any better.

It is a crime that we do not have a definite department in every college and in every high school to teach the prevention of disease and how to live properly. It is a crime that our labels, on what we eat, drink, or smoke, do not show the information that they contain materials

38

detrimental to our health and could produce disease. It is a shame that we have not been taught how to live by conscience, that we don't know the difference between right and wrong in many instances. Judge Mosk of Los Angeles says that lawbreaking has become so common among so many people because the dollar is the paramount goal in the lives of most people.

We do not put the right value on human life. From a spiritual standpoint, the fundamentals are: to be our brother's keeper, and to do unto others as we would have them do unto us. There is no religious concept used when coffee and doughnuts are served, when fried foods are given to our family, when white flour and white sugar are given to our children. The dentists know a better way, every man in the healing profession knows a better way of taking care of one another. It seems to be more difficult to do the right thing than the wrong thing.

When we try to tell people there is a better way of doing things, that there is better food, then we are called a "faddist", "a nut", or "a quack". If one tries to give a suggestion for a person's higher good, he is told to mind his own business. A heavy heart is produced when you see your loved ones around you deliberately doing the wrong thing, some ignorantly because of lack of education. When a humanitarian comes along to lift his fellowmen, they pull him down. When someone gives a suggestion of how to prevent disease, how to keep in good health, how to maintain good health, they throw tomatoes at him. It has been truly said that the more truth you have, the more right you have within you, the more alone you go. Isn't it a travesty that in this day and age when so many people are welcome to educational material, who are surrounded with huge libraries, have access to papers exchanging ideas, have television to bring out other people's ideas, the thoughts of manufacturers and the thoughts of producers—yet, in spite of the availability of all this useful and helpful information, a good 60 % of all advertisements are absolutely detrimental to the human economy and to human welfare.

THE PLIGHT OF MAN

Man can break down a molecule,
but cannot unite humanity.

You'll never live long enough to make *all* the mistakes yourself, so you might as well learn by contemplating the plight of your fellow men who ignored the warning. Look well at the mistakes he has made and avoid them.

It has been estimated that 80 % of the citizens of the United States are constipated and have spent something like 100 million dollars on laxatives during the last ten years. Now, isn t that enough money to spend just to learn that drug store laxatives are not the cure for constipation? There is something radically wrong with our training when we spend 9 million dollars a year for aspirin. That's a lot of headaches, especially when 90 % of them are unnecessary. They are due to our lack of knowledge in right living.

We must take time to meditate upon these vitally important things, to replace them with constructive ideas, and have our children join us. That is the best life insurance provision you can leave them, the best inheritance they can receive from their parents, together, of course, with a spiritual self-realization. This will insure their chances of maturing with greater understanding and compassion for their fellowmen. Also, it will insure their chances to have healthy, vigorous flesh, to be free of headaches, constipation, and all the other physical scourges from A to Z listed in the medical dictionary. For what is our hyper-modern civilization worth if we wind up in hospitals, mental institutions and jails? The population of these institutions is steadily increasing. We are continuously building more and larger structures for these purposes. Is that a credit to man? Have we not strayed away and become separated from the original plan for us? Where are we going? Where are we bound for? At this rate, our inevitable goal is ignoble extinction.

Turn on your IMAGINATION POWER and think upon the plight of the man who has the most wonderful peach orchard. For years this orchard has been the pride and joy of his heart. The peaches are organically grown and they are colorful and luscious—peaches ripened on the tree to be eaten the same day they are picked. He puts them into a box—not four or five days, or a week ahead of time when they are quite green—at the moment they are fit for human consumption. These crates of peaches could be the finest to be found in ANY store, ANYWHERE, yet he could not sell them. There is a law or ordinance that says every peach sold in a store must be of uniform size. When his perfectly-grown peaches are so much as an eighth of an inch smaller than that specified by law, they are declared unfit. Every box of peaches, even though properly grown and beautiful with the blush of natural perfection, is, according to this law, fit only to be fed to pigs.

Meanwhile, in the orchard across the fence from his, the peach grower is doing a land-office business. This orchard is complying with the law by growing peaches the size demanded; it does not matter that they are not grown organically. He does not use the proper fertilizer, and sprays his peaches so heavily with DDT that the birds will not cross the fence to taste them. The man-made law places the grower of the healthy peach in a predicament. To make a living, to make money to carry on, he is obliged to stop growing his peaches in the proper way — nature's way. He is forced to grow them under abnormal conditions, spraying and fertilizing his soil so that it is no longer fit to grow healthy fruit, only the kind the law demands.

Without intending to involve politics in this discussion of nutrition, I but present the peach grower's problem as an illustration of how the modern way of doing things is contrary to the law of nature — be it growing peaches of identical size or manufacturing too much white flour. Incidentally, nature's laws cannot be repealed; ignored, yes, but they cannot be taken off the books.

"City Jitters" Identified as New Disease
By George Getze (Times Science Writer)

PHILADELPHIA — Scientists here are discussing a new disease — "urbophrenia".

The scary-looking word can be loosely translated as "the city jitters", according to I. H. Kornblueh, medical director of the Department of Physical Medicine at the University of Pennsylvania.

Urbophrenia scars both the body and the mind of people who live in modern cities, spending nine-tenths of their time inside houses, air-conditioned cars and office buildings or factories.

Brains Get Lazy

They get nervous, their muscles get flabby from lack of exercise, and their brain gets lazy because of the wearisome monotony of their inside existence.

And the relaxing and sedating effects of nature do not get a chance to restore such city-dwellers to the health of surroundings more normal to mankind, Dr. Kornblueh said.

Los Angeles, with its individual house and back and front yards filled with geraniums, palm trees, and grass— even crab grass—has fewer sufferers from urbophrenia than most of the big cities of Europe and the eastern United States, it was suggested.

MODERN URBAN LIFE

In order to feed these increasing millions of city dwellers, a new approach to agriculture had to be envisaged. Those with an eye to selfish gain quickly saw a golden opportunity. Production was speeded up at the expense of quality. When the geographical frontier came to an end, urban areas encroached more and more on fields under cultivation. Every means of stretching food—from forcing production with the aid of artificial fertilizers and making war on anything threatening a total harvest, to inventing ways for the use of every possible by-product so that "nothing was left of the hog but the squeal," storage and preservation to the nth degree, and the transformation of vital products into puffed up "nothingness" or paper-thin, airy delusion—was perpetrated on it. Are these inventions as the writer of the Book of Ecclesiastes observes, causing man to affect his understanding of his true nature?

Man forgot that he could not forever reap harvest after harvest from the Good Earth without returning to her recompense in kind. With the depletion of the fertility of the soil there came the process of nature to destroy the land's inferior products, and upon man's crops descended an attack of insects which threatened to destroy the fruits of his labors. Science came to the rescue. She improved upon Nature, and we now have fruits and vegetables of every variety, huge and beautiful to the eye. But unseen and for long unsuspected are the residues of poisonous insect sprays and artificial fertilizers. Farmers' continual dumping onto the land tons and tons of fertilizer is not "replenishing the earth". Though designed to restore certain mineral elements to the soil, these inorganic materials merely stimulate a quick, unnatural growth in plants. We see a giant peach and we bite into it eagerly. But on every side nowadays comes the disillusioned cry, "Fruit doesn't taste like it used to!" How could it? And how also can it nourish our bodies adequately, when the bio-chemical elements we require are so sadly deficient in such foods? Yet still, instead of scientifically composting the residue from the huge quantities of raw materials, and the wastes from the millions of eating houses throughout the land, that which is not used to force-fatten the pig— an undesirable meat, at best—continues to constitute an endless problem in urban development.

It is very hard to maintain a degree of physical vitality high enough for complete well-being when living the modern urban life with its emphasis on automation, door-to-door transportation, push-button homes and indoor-centered interests. Because of our lack of exercise and our "citified" jobs, while other "less fortunate" peoples retain their physical hardihood, we are becoming a nation of the weak. There isn't even incentive to develop our higher potentials. We are sitting back and allowing our thinking to be taken over by robots. More and more capable electronic brains are doing it infinitely faster and more accurately. About the only opportunity for the use of a man's skill is in the continuing invention of these wizards! The tendency towards "soft" living is carried over to the foods we eat. Flabby internal muscles can no longer handle coarse natural foods; teeth made to enjoy chewing are crumbling structures or completely artificial, perverted palates crave the soft, smoother, lightness of refined foods. All of these factors have their effects upon the health and stamina of a people.

To compensate for the unhealthy conditions prevalent in city life, many people try to get out into the country whenever they can. But though we may still love the great out-of-doors, the places which have not been touched by the diabolic practices of man—where creatures of the wild may still be seen—are dwindling away. Pesticides and chemically polluted waters are fast destroying wildlife even in remote areas. Even unscrupulous sportsmen who have little understanding of the value of the lower orders of life and their place in the natural scheme of things take their toll. We are told of increasing demands to open these areas to commercial interests that people may come to develop them or bring them under cultivation. How will we educate our people into a deep appreciation of the beauty of nature in endless variety—for life itself—if we fail to preserve areas to which we may go to "get away from it all"?

SOFT LIVING IS OUR DOWNFALL

Continuing with his discussion of the Cuban situation, President Kennedy said, "Together we must build a hemisphere where freedom can flourish and where any free nation under outside attack can be assured that all our resources stand ready to respond to a request for assis--tance."

The same principle applies in the treatment and cure of disease. We must be conscious of and determined to maintain an internal power of resistance stronger than all germ life. To support such a state of health, it is necessary to provide the organism with the proper materials for building and repair. Only then will it not succumb to attacks which may be made upon it or fall victim to the stresses and tensions of life. Can we accept the challenge which the President presented? Our national survival, he explains, may depend upon it. "No greater task faces this nation or this administration. No other challenge is more deserving of our every effort and energy. For too long we have fixed our eyes on traditional military needs, on armies prepared to cross borders or missiles poised for flight. Now it should be clear that this is no longer enough —that our security may be lost piece by piece, country by country without the firing of a single missile or the crossing of a single border."

A nation is no stronger than the people of which it is comprised. The state of health of each individual may be a factor more necessary to our survival than we realize. The Russian people as a whole do not have the highly developed civilization with its accompanying luxury that the American people have. But we are killing ourselves with this very civilization and luxury. Dr. Paul Dudley White, former President Eisenhower's physician, stated in a medical convention that the luxury which man enjoys can be the very thing that produces so much of the heart trouble and ill health we have today. He talked about our young men not having the strength and power youth used to have because the type of work that exists for many is sedentary. Automobiles carry us to and fro, eliminating proper exercise; the life of ease which we seek is detrimental to our physical health. Eating degenerated, man-handled, devitalized foods, over-indulging in desserts, and between-meal snacking are not habits building strength.

It has been said that the downfall of France came when, because of war production, they brought the people in from the farms to the cities in organized groups to work in the factories, build fortifications and guns and munitions to preserve their country. They came to enjoy the sensual luxuries of life which eventually were the major contributing factor to their downfall.

With this picture in the background, we can see that America, too, can lose its vital force, its brain power and its health if we continue pursuit of the luxury life we enjoy today. The huge city developments, organized manufacturing methods and mechanized means of production can all contribute to America's downfall. One of the most important things we must be aware of is that man's inventions can so tamper with our food supply—that vital life-line which keeps us well and healthy—as to destroy us. Man's inventions have already changed foods from their natural state—the garden state which the peasant and simple peoples of the earth still enjoy if left to their own way of life—into a mechanized state. Our foods have been processed and devitalized, then fortified, preserved, colored and flavored. Consuming these over a period of time results in a prolonged deficiency which will sap our vital energies. Some of the drugs and preservatives used will cause irritated nervous systems. In the same way our coffee breaks can produce liver disturbances. Stimulation without compensation for regaining vital energies can lead to depletion.

DEVITALIZED FOOD ON THE INCREASE

Recent magazine articles tell us that we have some 3,000 packaged foods on our grocery shelves today, and that within five years we will have 15,000 items. If these contained fresh, vital, untampered foods, they would unquestionably be for man's good, but we know that the processing and devitalization to which they are subjected degenerate the natural functionings of the human organism.

A short time ago I listened to a young lady telling her plans for her future life. She said that she planned to have a career, to be married and have a family. In fact, she had many ideas about things she hoped to accomplish. When asked how she could have a career and a family at the same time, she said that with TV dinners and all the prepared foods available today, you no longer had to know how to cook. It was all done for you.

The average kitchen today is another weak link in the chain of health of every man, woman and child. We associate the process of "brainwashing" with the activities of an opposing political ideology, but there is probably a worse type of brainwashing going on among us that directly affects the great majority of our people. That is what is being done in the food business.

CHOLESTEROL

Cholesterol is a normal substance found in all bodies; however, there is such a thing as having too large an organ, too much sugar in the blood, and it is also possible to have too much cholesterol. When we have an excess amount of cholesterol in the blood, it can be deposited in the arteries, causing a hardened tissue that cannot physiologically function well. This cholesterol is made internally by chemical changes that occur within the body. This is called an endogenous source, and it comes also from what is called unsaturated fats taken in the food, which is called exogenous source. In other words, an excess amount of cholesterol can be formed in the body from internal means or from the foods that we take externally. There is a chemical process called lipid metabolism going on in the body.

We need a certain amount of the fatty substances for the maintenance of our body's health, and it takes a lipid metabolism to bring about the changes for the proper development of the fatty substances for our bodies. They say that when we have above the normal level of cholesterol in the blood, it can be associated with disease of the arteries known as arteriosclerosis.

The inside coat of an artery is roughened, and little flat plaques form on it when the blood cholesterol is high. When these little flat plaques settle in the arteries they attract blood which sticks to these areas forming clots. Clots are something to avoid in the blood stream, because they obstruct circulation. When these clots form in the vital organs, we can be in real trouble. When scientists find this blood cholesterol high, they try to bring it to a normal level. When people reduce in weight, usually the blood cholesterol comes down. In most cases we find that a change of cholesterol can take place when we make a change in the diet.

In the Journal of the Medical Association there was a discussion reported by Doctor Kinsell of California in which he gave three diets. The first and most stringent contains no animal fat. Necessary proteins are supplied not by meat, but by milk without fat, cereals, nuts and vegetables. Later they can give fish, fowl, and then liver is added. Finally, in the third stage, they use lean beef, veal, lamb and eggs. However, I do think that we should be more strict in cases where we have definitely developed this cholesterol in the body.

The Trappist Monks in Canada are a group of vegetarians who have brothers called the St. Benedictine Monks in Georgia, who live on a good deal of the meat products. They have tested both of these orders and find that the vegetarian order does not have cholesterol deposits in their arteries or have a cholesterol level in their blood stream like those we find in the St. Benedictine Monks of the south. Every single one, on the average, of the whole group of the St. Benedictines, had a high level of cholesterol. I do believe that this demonstrates that possibly meat can be one of the things bringing on high cholesterol in these people.

I believe that cholesterol can be formed in the body by having many of the fatty foods of animal origin, such as eggs, butter, milk, cream, as well as the fatty meats and fish. The average doctor hasn't practiced nutrition enough to know just how he can control this in his patients, but we who have used dietetic control in cholesterol cases for many years find that diet works very well. The Heart Department of the National Institute of Health in Washington proved that certain key substances that are found in hormones are lacking which break up the fat foods in persons suffering from these diseases. Where some cannot handle excess sugars, others cannot handle fats. Many of the patients who are suffering from a rise in blood cholesterol are not exercising properly; therefore there is a lack of oxidation, and the foodstuffs have become so rich that the body isn't well enough to take care of them. Heavy cholesterol in most people is caused by rich living.

For some reason or another, people in this day and age seem to think that fats are needed in order to keep warm or to build the body weight, etc., but this is not always true. A thin body is likely to be desired much more than an overweight one. It is said that the larger the waistline, the shorter the life line. It is well that we avoid overweight and the many fats, oils and creams in our diet that cause this excess. I believe that cholesterol is a disease of civilization. Greens are especially good in aiding the metabolism of fats, and most of us do not have enough of these green leaves in salads and other foods. Many of us would be much better off if we would take the vegetable fats in place of the animal fats. We believe that cholesterol is the result of poor living which goes hand in hand with aging and hardening of the arteries.

To decrease cholesterol excess, it might be well to go on a meat-free diet for a while, eliminating the use of concentrated fats and oils. If oils are used, make sure that they are unheated. Never have fried foods, use lots of salads and lots of green foods. Have green teas, such as comfrey tea, dandelion tea; also use a lot of whey in your diet which is high in sodium and has a heavy dissolving ability. Lecithin in the diet helps to break down the cholesterol content of the arteries and in the blood.

Cocktails made of celery juice, cucumber juice or spinach—in place of the civilized popular cocktails at the bar—will break down the cholesterol content of the arteries. Find a good healthy way to live, and especially be interested in keeping the liver in good active order. Find exercises that keep the liver in a good active condition. A sedentary occupation can be conducive to building cholesterol in the body. We must find a way of changing our lives, a way to balance our daily routine.

Let me bring out another interesting thing. Birds have a

heart rate of 120 beats per minute; horses only 35 and an elephant is down to 25 beats per minute. Do you suppose the heart rate in an elephant could be the same as in a man? No. This all goes to show that nature takes good care of all of us. In an infant, the heartbeat is twice that of an adult. Nature has taken care of that also.

INSIDIOUS SUICIDE

We may be frightened by the prospects of sudden death in an atomic blast; perhaps we have sneaking fears of the effects of radioactivity on our future children; we may be horrified to think that many will be sterile as a result of the rays—but now we are told of an even greater menace, a slow yet relentless destroyer of life on the planet, for what could be more totally destructive than the deadening of our emotional desires? It seems that if we survive the holocaust, an insidious death of civilization will follow. We may escape with our 'lives', but we will be beset with intense nervous disorders from shock, listlessness and emotional instability. We will be creatures with no desires. Male and female love will be physically impossible. The glands will not function properly.

In World War II, the Nazis used X rays to sterilize large numbers of subjected peoples. What a puny method compared to our modern hydrogen bomb—and there is talk of even deadlier types—from a mere few hundred square miles of area affected, now whole nations will be within the contamination of one explosion.

When the pall of smoke clears away and the living gather themselves up out of the debris to reckon up their futures, what will be the prospects from a race survival angle? Primarily, the reproductive glands will have been affected; many will be completely sterile. Nervous disorders are always known to reduce desire—and nervous disorders will be rife in those who escape most of the radiation. Those women still with normal desires will face the possibilities of later psychological frigidity if the men they love fail to respond because of glandular damage.

Observation of those already subjected to radioactivity indicates the development of a new disease "tabes" which affects the spinal cord, often leaving the victim romantically indifferent. The prostate gland is very vulnerable to radiation damage. Men affected with the resulting inflammation will feel little inclination for love making. A similar inflammation occurs in the suprarenal glands which produce a secretion closely allied to the male hormone, but connection with sex has not yet been verified.

Reports on the Nazi sterilization victims show a ray-type of total castration. In animals, this alters the body line, makes a wild creature tame, easy-going and manageable. We are already familiar with the timid, high-voiced and hairless eunuchs of Far Eastern courts.

Another hazard awaits us. A major 'flu' epidemic will probably develop. Those near the site of a nuclear explosion will suffer damage to their natural immunization mechanism which protects them against the influenza virus. Tests conducted by Dr. James Quilligan at Loma Linda University Laboratory, Los Angeles (supported by the U.S. Atomic Energy Commission) with mice already show that the nearer the center of radio activity, the more rapidly grow the influenza viruses, and the more persistently they last, because the antibodies protecting against the influenza fail to reach "good" levels in the bloodstream.

The days when a mother mourned the loss of a son in a foreign battle are gone. If there is another war, you will be in the middle of it, I will be in it. We have our own little wars going on against poisoned foods and greedily-robbed soils, but let us not lose sight of the giant monster, and pray for Peace in Our Time.

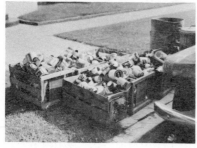

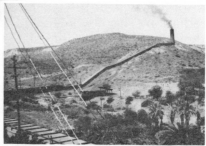

Chapter 5

I Came, I Saw.....

The subject of longevity has been of quite an interest to me for some time. As you get older you start thinking about it. I've been studying this for some years now.

The first thing I did was read a book on how to live to be 100 years of age. I thought I ought to find the man who wrote it. When I met him, I found he was only 26 years old!

I started gathering material as I went along. I saw in the paper where a man in Los Angeles was 106 years of age. I knocked on his door and asked him if he was that man, and he said "Yes." Then I asked him if there were any secrets to living that long. He said, "Yes. Just keep breathing."

I don't feel that just old age is what most people want to attain. We must have good health also. When I visited India I noticed that the people living in poverty don't seem to be bothered by it. They think it's part of life. They die at a very young age because about 80% of the population is starving for protein. The average life span at the time of my first visit was 21. In the last few years it's been going up to 31,32,33 as they use more antibiotics and build more hospitals to treat the children who otherwise would die very young. I wonder when I look at these people just how long you have to live to put in a good life. Have they lived a good life? Just what can I learn from them?

Traveling around the world I became interested in the cultures of various people and what they did that enabled them to live that way. Each country seems to offer something outstanding. It may be three things, it may be many things. I'd like to go through these countries with you and share some of the highlights we found.

One of the first essential factors we see is that everybody has to make a living. Everybody was born to do something— born, more or less, to serve. There's a lot of happiness in serving, although the average person today doesn't necessarily feel that way. I really feel that you'll never be happy unless you're helping other people. Your success from a health standpoint or a happiness standpoint comes from uplifting others. This is the most important Key in every country. Whether it be in a family, a community or a group, people have to help and serve one another. You can't live by yourself. There is no reason to live by yourself. You probably could live a long life by yourself, but for what reason? I'm sure it would be a very selfish one.

In this country we think a great deal about retiring. We think about what we can do, where we are going, and what we are fit for, and what we can accomplish when we get to retirement age. If you look around, you'll see that it doesn't matter what you accomplish after the age of 60 or 65 anymore. Nobody wants you. It seems like they've put you on a shelf. Yet, the wisest man is living after 60, 70, or 80. I've learned my best lessons from old men.

My greatest nature cures and the wisdom they taught me came from old John Harvey Kellogg before he died; Old Dr. Victor Rocine, at the age of 90; and old Dr. Tilden in Denver before he died in his late 80's.

These men who have lived a long life should have something to pass along to the next generation and children who are yet to come. I don't think we live long enough today to pass on knowledge to our next generation. We have a lot of experiences, but we don't have the wisdom yet to go along with them. We haven't been able to make good decisions because of our experiences. Most of us are still experiencing when we die—experiencing poor health, in most cases. Most of us don't even know how to take care of ourselves financially, and many die poor. We've got to learn to live with finances or without finances. I feel that living a long life is not good enough in most cases, but a good life lived is long enough.

The average person goes through the various levels of life, one period after another, without really living a good life. I don't feel sorry for the man who has died; I feel sorry for the man who has never lived. How many moments can you look back on and say, "Didn't we have a wonderful time?" "Wasn't that a lovely evening?" Many people can only count these experiences on one hand as they go through life, and that is because most people just exist. I hear this all the time from patients: "I'm just a housewife." "I'm just a farmer" "I'm just a mechanic." There should be something wonderful in all these jobs—unless you make something humdrum out of it. You must find a meaningful and joyous way to live.

One thing I know, you'll never be well unless you're happy. Have a good life while you are living.

I question this idea of living just a long life. Who wants to be just live tissue? Who wants just two good bowel movements a day? Who wants just a good heartbeat, but no love in their heart? This idea of living a long life is not the real key. The key is to be known by your accomplishments.

What have you done in life? What have you given to this world that is of a good nature? What have you shared with others? Is this a better place for your being here? Are you leaving it for better or for worse? These are your decisions to make.

I've learned in going through these countries that we have to look at longevity from a spiritual, mental and physical standpoint. A lot of people have the idea that food is everything. They think diet is everything.

From Great Britain I learned that a man cannot be overweight and live long. A man who is 20 lbs. underweight lives the longest life according to insurance statistics, and a person who does not work all his life does not live long.

There are some people who are so spiritually inclined that the physical body doesn't mean a thing. Everything is soul development. Buddhism, Hinduism, many oriental or eastern philosophies tell us we have an astral life that is much more important than this life here. There are many who are living an afterlife now. They have an idea that whatever they do now is earning them a place in heaven. Even the Christian philosophy will tell you that, too. Your rewards will be in heaven. There will be a "rest beyond the river." They offer something very nice later on, but right now is an important time in our lives. You are living in Eternity right now. There is only one life. The inner life is very important.

There is one thing I've learned from visiting these old men more than anything else, and that is that they are living a life of prevention. They are not walking into disease. We haven't grasped this yet. Doctors have waiting rooms, waiting for you to have a sickness. Nine billion dollars is being spent on hospitals in the next nine months. They're waiting for you. They know you are coming. We have institutions to match our sicknesses today.

The real old men have another type of institution—it's nature. It's natural surroundings where the environment is clean and wholesome—a place where a person can live a long life and not find himself dwindling away.

All these wise old men consider the soil "Mother Earth." Mother Earth takes care of you from a food standpoint, from a shelter standpoint, and for the future. All of these people used natural water. Not particularly distilled water, but natural mountain water. They live at a certain climate—a mild climate—and at certain altitudes.

These people have plenty of exercise. It's in their work. Why is it among these elderly people that the women die first? In the U.S. women live 8 years longer than men. But among these very elderly people of the Balkans, Russia, Turkey, Armenia, Bulgaria and Rumania, we find the women dying 20 and 30 years before the men. Right about the age of 70 the women come inside. They go into the house and put on their slippers. They are walking on a hard, flat surface in flat-soled shoes and their legs do not get the proper amount of exercise daily. The men were out in the fields with the sheep and gardening all day. Leg muscles are developed by climbing in the mountains and hills, and are a great source of pride to these men.

We have a wonderful exercise for the legs at our Ranch here, and that is walking in the hills. You can't walk on a level surface around here and this helps to take care of the legs. Walk in these hills and enjoy the beautiful surroundings!

Many who lived a long life in Turkey were those kicking on carpets to clean them all day long. I'm convinced that leg activities brought the men the long life and the women the short life. Whether we are men or women, many of us are sitting too much. Heart trouble comes from this—also from driving cars too much. We don't straighten out our legs and we don't develop our leg muscles. This is one of the great Keys to keeping us well.

Using Iridology, I found there were not any extreme cases of senility. This is an anemic condition of the brain and is not found with these old people. They have wonderful memories and can recall incidents of a hundred years ago as well as something that happened twenty-five years ago. Their minds are alert and they can answer questions immediately. They do not have to stop and think it over, they are right on the ball.

This is one of the main factors that comes from having good leg muscles. Without these good leg muscles, you cannot force the blood back into the body again. If you want to get blood back into the head area, you do it through the legs. This is why I believe walking to be so helpful.

We have spent a lot of time researching information on these elderly people. We read a lot of books, listened to a lot of tales given to us by people at gas stations, markets, hotels; and of course we sought after a lot of these people in different countries.

When we met these people we found they were not aware of the qualities that actually gave them a long life and good health, because they had never travelled or met people outside of their own country, or even their own village. They did not know how people were living in other parts of the world.

I thought that after I had the figures showing that the average person in New Zealand lived to the age of 79, I would find the oldest person in the world living there. The oldest person I could find was Granny Nga, a native Maori woman of 123 years of age. Her name, when translated means "Tree that never dies."

We found Granny Nga to be quite spry. She smoked a pipe, had an extremely good sense of humor and liked to sing. She sang to us and told us about the boys and girls in her younger days. She felt very well indeed and thought she was ready for another 123 years.

One of the Keys I learned from Granny Nga was that when she was having troubles as far as her body was concerned— when she felt ill, had a fever, or had a lack of energy—she always went down to the river. It was by taking cold baths there in the river that she felt better.

I feel that this Key of using water is a very important one. This is because the Polynesian race, of which Granny Nga was a member, lived in a climate that threw off a lot of the sodium salts and kept this kind of person in a higher temperature than those elderly people that we will discuss later. These people also lived in a hot climate, but ate many of the fruits that were grown there and were high in sodium to replace the sodium salts they would perspire away.

While in New Zealand, I could definitely see one of the Keys to their long life was that they considered their weekends, from Friday night to Monday morning, a holiday time. They would go out on the beaches, go out in their boats, go swimming, and this was the most important part of their weekly routine. In fact, every school in New Zealand has a swimming pool. Great Olympic champions have come from New Zealand. These people appreciate their mountains and oceans and use them. There are more yachts per person than any other place else in the world. People really enjoy life there!

Their tempo is at a moderate pace where they never wear themselves out. You can almost see it expressed in their automobiles. Some of them are running old Fords and Chevrolets, all in good condition. They've been off our roads a long time, and we battered the devil out of them. But New Zealanders can take care of their cars and themselves. They keep busy but they do not overdo. They do not abuse their bodies in their activities.

Although they excel in the practice of the Key of Rest and Relaxation, there are other Keys which haven't been up to what I would call a point of efficiency that could give them a longer life than they already have.

Most of the people of New Zealand are fit, but they do have one outstanding health problem. They have the poorest teeth of any country in the world. Although the average person lives until the age of 79 he doesn't have all the calcium he needs. Calcium is our long life element. I do believe, though, that the amount of sunshine they have, their ability to enjoy life and relax at any easy tempo allows them to live a long life.

Their food situation is not the best. The balance in the diet is not the best. I don't believe their soil in some cases is the best, but in many places in New Zealand it is beautiful. They have beauty, they have harmony, they have many of the Keys working for them to give them a good, healthy life.

MAORI WISDOM
from
New Zealand

- Youth talks age teaches
- Little dogs make the most noise
- Wishing never filled a game bag
- A fine foodhouse doesn't fill itself
- No one needs help to get into trouble
- An idle young man—an unhappy old man
- A bad thing usually costs a lot
- A pigeon won't fly into a wide open mouth
- Great griefs are silent

- The widest mouth has the widest grave
- Time to dream when you are dead
- Chase two Moas—catch none
- Never be late to a battle to win it
- An obedient wife commands her warrior
- Beauty won't fill the puku (stomach)
- A wise man knows pain
- One rotten fish, one fresh fish—two rotten fish
- The God of evil and the God of fear are good friends
- A warrior without courage has a blunt taiaha (spear)
- The brighter the clearing the darker the shadows
- Today's meal is better than tomorrow's tangi (feast)
- No twigs on the fire—no flame

In India they have the Keys working for them very strongly in the religious and spiritual areas; and they too have worked with color and harmony and beauty. Their philosophy is very advanced, but I believe they have been very short in the available foods. In many places we found they did not have the climate conducive to a healthy life. The food and the soil, I feel, have been their greatest detriments in having a long life and, of course, the proper amount of proteins. To balance life we must combine the physical, mental and spiritual.

I believe they have been short on the physical side of life, but this aspect was developed well in Sri Aurobindo's ashram where they exercised daily and ate a balanced diet with enough protein. Of course, I realize the purpose of the yoga exercises is to make the body a humble servant to the mind and the spirit. It provides a state of inner peace and the ability to relax at will.

I travelled to the Northern part of India, into Darjeeling, and became acquainted with the terraced method of farming. It was here that I heard about the "Valley of Eternal Youth"; and I knew that in my seeking I would someday find this Valley if I kept on with the search constantly and long enough.

I have gone to the South Seas and experienced the therapeutic value of nature's beauty; the philosophy and the life style of the Tahitian people left a deep impression on me. It was there that I felt serenity and tranquility, and it was there that I discovered the art of living. They really enjoyed their dances, and of course the Tahitian "shake-up" is a wonderful thing for that lazy liver. They knew what joy was and what a happy moment was. I discovered that the life span of these people has been shortened since the missionaries talked them into wearing clothes. They used the sunshine to help hold the calcium in their bodies.

They use coconuts there for just about everything. They wean a baby using coconut milk. They also use it to set bones. The green coconut, soft on the inside, has a delicious taste. But I didn't find the long-lived people in Tahiti. There used to be long lived people here and in Hawaii. Captain Cook said that the Hawaiians used to carry 300 and 400 lbs. on their backs from the ship. After they began eating the white flour and white sugar products they couldn't carry those loads the next time he docked. This shows that the natural foods were giving them the strength and power and energy to live and work as they did.

I also wondered if perspiring didn't contribute to their shorter life. The salty taste of perspiration is sodium—the youth element. It is stored in the joints and stomach. I know if you wear out and throw out all that sodium in the body it is difficult to be healthy and well. It was here that I discovered the value of walking in the sand to strengthen the smaller muscles of the legs. It was here that I realized what Paul Dudley White said, that we die from our feet up. And as Bernarr McFadden said, the exercise that would help our legs is the thing that would keep our brain alive. For it was here, as both of these men showed me, that we began to force the blood uphill. To have a good circulation from the feet meant a good circulation in the brain areas. In days to come, when I would meet these old men, I could see that they had a good circulation and good brain activity because they took care of their legs.

It was in the Virgin Islands that I saw that music was very necessary to hold people together, and they were going to have music no matter what happened. They had their drums taken away from them that they had used in centuries past in Africa; but they developed a music from the steel drums that were left there from the war that carried oil and gasoline. Music was part of their soul. It is part of everyone that I met wherever I travelled. I saw that their slow pace of living and their mild temper traits were outstanding in giving them their good health and what long life they did have.

When we went to Peru I noticed that in the higher altitudes the people had a higher blood count than any other place in the world. I recognize what Dr. Rollier meant when he said that his patients got well better in the Alps than anywhere else because of the clear sunshine that came to the mountains. It was both the altitude and the sight of the sun that gave these people a wonderful control of the calcium in their bodies, a healing element. Here is where sores would heal best and where people from all over the world were getting what was called the "Sun-Cure."

I saw in Switzerland where goat cheese was used and many of the sanitariums were using the whey cheese for special arthritic conditions to keep the joints active. In Germany we recognize that the health spas take over the biggest part of the countryside. Beauty abounds in the hills, but the wonderful water treatments practiced there build up the circulation of the body; and this goes along with the idea that to just have a good bloodstream and not a good circulation makes it difficult to have good health.

When we went to Worishofen we watched this technique that was developed by Father Kneipp, a Catholic priest, in the late 1800's. It was used in the entire community. There were over 4,000 homes in this community that you could go to and get these cures. There barefooted walks in grass after the Kneipp baths, and walking through wading pools of cold water, was certainly effective in developing a good circulation in the lower extremities of the body and for the good of the whole body. Father Kneipp claimed that the blood pressure normalized itself, and the activity in the heart and circulatory system was improved.

They have treatments for people to walk in cold water up to their knees. There is a central park where every morning groups of people take the water treatment. They lift up their knees while walking in the water trough; then they come out and run through the park of beautiful green grass. It's cold and damp and dewy. You don't just stand there and say "aah," you really move! After the bath you dry off by moving around, and circulation is stimulated by walking in the cold grass.

I use the Kneipp cure at the Hidden Valley Ranch and my patients tell me that about the third day they don't have cold feet when they go to bed at night.

I know this to be true: when your toes become blue and start turning up, things are getting serious. One of the first things we should do in taking care of our health is to work with the legs and feet. This is one of the finest keys to keep living a long time.

It was Dr. Alexis Carrell who startled the world when he announced that he had conducted experiments that proved that tissue cells can be immortal. He had fed a chicken's heart on egg yolk protein and was able to keep it alive for over 29 years. I saw the value of protein in just this one experience. In Heliconia, Columbia, I saw an entire community that was affected by not having enough protein in their diet, and the average person in this community was dying at the age of 30. Yet by adding a soy bean milk powder this was changed completely. I found that the value of protein in the diet was a necessary factor to consider.

The Scandinavians took care of their skin through exercise and sauna bath rituals.

I learned something in Denmark that bothered me. They have more suicides than any other country in the world. They also claim to use more artificial fertilizer and sprays on their fruits and vegetables than any other country in the world also, and I wondered if there was a relation between the two. I was looking for everything.

Denmark has a recipe for one of the highest foods in calcium, a soup called "Grunco." This is a soup made of greens, kale and barley.

In Finland they use a lot of rye. Rye develops muscle in the body. I began to contrast that with countries that use so much wheat. Wheat builds fat; rye builds muscle. Out of Finland we have the greatest Olympic runners we have ever had. Many of these runners have probably learned that rye is one of the greatest of all our grains.

It was in Lourdes, France, that I saw where faith and hope was practiced to such an extent that peace and harmony prevailed throughout the city. It permeated the atmosphere and was expressed by all who attended the services. Sixteen thousand people a day were taken to the shrine in wheelchairs and many were cured with faith alone. I was interested in the miracle of life and how much faith do we really need to produce a miracle in our healing. But it was well to see what the mind could do and what the spiritual attitude could accomplish in life. Lourdes is a living monument to faith, where all mankind can unite in brotherhood and prayer. Love and beauty came forth in these elderly people I met and I found it was their philosophy, and not just the food, that recharged many a person's inner self. Without that, many felt empty, going through life just a physical being.

Beauty was so effectively brought out in nature; and as these people met the naturalness of life they found the upliftment Francis Bacon described when he said, "A walk in the garden is the purest of human pleasures; it is the greatest refreshment to the spirit of man." The aesthetic value of beauty is a necessary ingredient in a well-balanced life. I saw love expressed in many ways throughout the world, and a lack of love in the family circle or a lack of social acceptance in the community life altered a person's hormone level and brought about changes in the nervous system, causing a generalized susceptibility to diseases.

I saw where a good marriage benefited a person's health and helped produce a long life, while other marriages could break down a person and produce a short life. This probably explains why the death rate of divorced men is 3 to 5 times higher than that of married men the same age.

In my spiritual quest I traveled into the Yucatan peninsula of lower Mexico and saw how the Mayans had lived 3,000 years before Christ through many hardships. The most important thing in their lives was the sun, rain and corn; and they looked up to them as gods that were most essential to their lives. Their culture was very important to them, and they left messages in their hieroglyphics. They built temples to the turtles, and they had wells of sacrifice and halls of fame and astronomical observatories. Yes, they had an interesting life that they lived; and whether it produced a long life and a healthy one is hard to say. Yet again, they had things they believed were most important to them. Their habits included living in the sun, bathing, and using the love temples, the basis of their love culture. I wonder if we couldn't learn from these past civilizations. In these past cultures religion and learning were very closely intertwined.

They had their crafts and their gardening and their marketing; but we found that they were living a life close to nature, and body rejuvenation was very important to them. Agriculture was at the basis of their knowledge and the structure of their culture. Market scenes were brought to our attention in their hieroglyphics, and how the roads that passed these ancient buildings were lined with markets years ago.

In South America, we saw where the Spaniards had entered Cuzco, and we were, of course, startled by the sight of the gold plated buildings. They stripped these palaces and temples of their treasures and melted down the gold. Very little is left now of these Incan art objects.

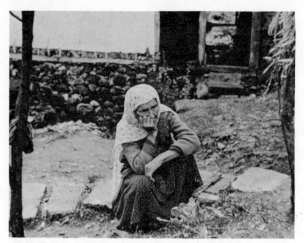

Candelaria Hill, 125 years, Central America. She lives deep in the mountains with her 80 year old daughter.

This Mexican man, 100 years of age, lives a very simple life on the desert plains. He had lived a rugged life as a farmer so his life was filled with physical adventure, giving him the exercise and circulation he needed.

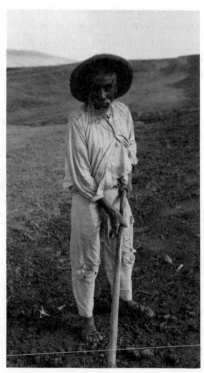

At Machu Piccu, the "lost city in the sky" that was built on top of a mountain, people had to be of good physical development in order to live there. They had to have knowledge and they had to have wisdom to bring water to the high mountain peaks. We found their terraces where they preserved the soil and took care of every bit of available growing ground because they needed food for the continuation of life.

It was designed to be a completely self-sufficient city, and it served as a sanctuary for the royal family, religious leaders and the virgins of the sun. They had irrigation systems to carry the water from the highest peak down through delicate yet strong canals.

Thailand offered us a smile that certainly was unique in itself. It was a happy land, with many gentle, gracious people living there. This is part of a good life. Their dances were most beautiful and the music they played brought out a lovely dance, indeed. We have known for years that music had been used to treat mental illnesses; music has been used in many branches of the healing arts for stimulating the brain and activating nerve cells. Music can stimulate a man's inner self in such a way that it lifts him to his highest nature.

It was in Cambodia and in their ruins that we could see that there was a Master Mind working in the past. They put rocks together without mortar, or cement; yet they were so closely put together you could not see through them or put a knife between the rocks. They were soil people. They were close to the earth; they knew how to use what was around them to build and to construct.

I believe that India offered more to think about than any country in the world. It was the Taj Mahal, a memorial to love, that moved me most; and yet, again we saw poverty and many things of which people are not aware. We found riches there that would overwhelm you; yet we found those having the riches were lacking much that only the poor soil man possessed.

I spent time with the Dalai Lama of Tibet at his place in Northern India. He believes there is so much to life when we meditate and that through concentration one is able to develop many levels of consciousness that we couldn't develop otherwise. We went into the subject of prophecy and reincarnation; and there are some people who are so interested in this that it is part of their lives. Some people cannot have the best of health until they answer some of the questions they have been seeking for many years. Some people find complete satisfaction in this realm of living; and I am sure that the nervous system would be better for that type of philosophy. There are others who cannot go along with this philosophy and have to find satisfaction in another type of religion.

So there are religions for different kinds of people, for different levels of consciousness. As we seek, so shall we find.

It was at the River Ganges that we recognized the beautiful spirit people have towards the earth and the waters thereof, for the Indians look to the Ganges as the beginning of all life.

And it was in India we heard that during an epidemic 5,000 people died of cholera and 20,000 people died of the *fear* of cholera. Again, the philosophy of India can be overwhelming when we realize it has a scientific background. They have discovered today that fear can kill more people than war.

The high point of all my visits in India was my communication with Sai Baba of Puthaparti, in the southern part of India. He has millions of followers and he is truly an avator who many are finding more comfort and security in than in anything else. Sai Baba said that love is one of man's greatest Keys because "if you love all of God's creations then you love the God Force. Love God above all else and Love your neighbor as yourself. If you do that you will always find ways and means of helping each other." I do feel this man has control and dominion over not only himself, but others and his surroundings. He mentioned that in America we probably have a lot of money, but we also have a lot of comfort. "Money buys that comfort. We do not have that much comfort in this country, but we have contentment." And isn't contentment a necessary element in living a long life? I feel our spiritual attitude is very, very essential in living a full life.

He produced many miracles that awed the people who came there, and many need demonstrations before they believe. I saw him perform the miracle of materializing the vibhuti, the sacred ash, from an empty urn. It is said that this vibhuti endows one with prosperity and burns away sin, removes danger and increases one's spiritual splendor. He spent 15 minutes turning his hand around in the inside of a one-gallon brass urn, and brought out ashes constantly until they were many feet high on the floor. People used this vibhuti in little envelopes on their tongue to cure both mental and physical ailments. People certainly left with a warm glow in their hearts and a firm desire to carry out Sai Baba's message of love to one another.

It was at Sri Aurobindo's ashram that we saw the best example of a physical, mental and spiritual balance. We saw these people using more protein in their diet than the average Indian gets. We found that they gathered together and partook of exercise every day, such as swimming, wrestling, and tennis, which gave them beautiful bodies. It may be that you would not see this in any other part of India. It was here that they have a great ideal to start a new city, a city of peace, called Auroville. This moved me tremendously because today we need this so much, and man is looking for that Shangri-La—that ideal place—where all of humanity can come together and live as One. Here is the only place in the world where I saw that they were actually trying to live and practice in daily life that which is deepest in man's heart.

To see the mental and the spiritual qualities both being used in the various countries moved me tremendously, because some people are more interested in a spiritual manifestation than in anything else. I wondered about the work that the Fiji Islanders were engrossed in when they did the fire walking. Was it a mental thing? A spiritual thing? Or, was it hypnotism? I saw the control over the mind in walking on those hot coals, a thing that you possibly wouldn't do with the conscious mind.

I saw the value of trees in many countries; they are valuable shields against various pollutants. In smoggy times these trees would die out and pass away. I could see that these trees were man's best friend and that we had to take better care of them.

It was the trees in the Balkan States, especially the pine, that they call the sacred tree. It was for their life and health, it meant much to them. To destroy a tree was almost as bad as destroying the life of a person.

I have had a great interest in the soil, and in various parts of the world—especially in Peru—I saw many vegetables and fruits there. This is the food center of the world. Tomatoes originally came from Peru. We might think that potatoes come from Ireland, but they originally came from Peru. You have heard of lima beans; they came from Lima, Peru. They used herbs and had the most beautiful vegetables of any country in any part of the world.

Yet there are many things that are conducive to bringing on a long life. I wondered if it was mostly the soil; and in my investigation which I started many years ago when I started the Hidden Valley Health Ranch, I saw where vegetables were dependent upon the type of soil in which they were grown, and that you could change the vegetable life by changing the soil. I began to wonder if these elements in the soil would finally reach mankind and would dwarf him in his balance, or would interfere with his health.

I saw this occur in Guatemala, one of the most populated countries in South America. We find they don't have a long life span, yet their Indian communities are largely self-sustaining. I saw them selling all their protein and living more on starches and carbohydrates.

You can see an exaggerated example of a straight spine, a beautiful carriage, and a beautiful posture in South America and Central America where people, particularly the women, carry huge loads on their heads. Pots of water and food are carried. These people really walk straight, and I recognize that posture is one of those Keys we must have. I realized it when I met all the different elderly people, for I never found a bent-over old man.

When you travel around the world you see that finances have a different place of importance in various countries. Some barter for what they have and the talents they have put into this; others use money, and there are still others that if you enjoyed what they had, they would almost give it to you.

I had an unusual experience in South America where I bought an orange. It tasted so wonderful that I went back to buy the rest of them from the woman. There were 11 oranges left but she wouldn't sell them to me all at one time because she wouldn't have anything else to do the rest of the day if they were all sold.

In the Amazon I saw where the water washed away all the top soil. The DeColorado Indians were the least healthy of all the people I found in my travels throughout South America. They had extreme height where the pituitary gland wasn't well developed, and this was probably due to a lack of protein.

We also saw that they had pigeon chests and pronated ankles. Their bodies were developing rickets and had a lack of calcium. I wonder if this calcium lack in these people wasn't a main factor in developing the kind of bodies they had. I never saw this kind of body in the elderly people in Turkey, Bulgaria, Russia, Vilcabamba, etc.

I had one of my finest visits in regard to health and long life in the little town of Vilcabamba in Equador. It is a community where they say there is no heart trouble, and I found this to be true. Many of the elderly people there could run many blocks without tiring.

I went down to Ecuador where I saw a man of 143 years of age in the town of Vilcabamba. The town was very, very slow. You could walk down a street and nothing was happening. The first thing I said to Marie was that they don't move fast enough in this city to die. We found that they just don't wear themselves out.

We found a little old lady there who jogs 10 blocks every morning. People in this community never die of heart trouble. No high blood pressure or tension can be found here. I wondered if it was their tempo of life or just what it was. A man from one of the neighboring towns had a heart attack and came to this village. Within 3 days he no longer had any signs of his troubles; his whole body changed. His glands, heart and breathing changed. He was driving his car, one of the tires blew out and he got out of the car and pumped up the tire with a hand pump 250 times. Three days before he said he couldn't have pumped it once. He thought getting over this heart attack was wonderful because he was able to chase women again.

I became acquainted with a man of 140 years of age. I visited him in his home for awhile and asked him about any sickness. He said he had been sick—with pneumonia at the age of 104. I told him he must have gotten over it okay because he looked pretty good at age 140. He answered, "Oh, yes, I used some of the herbs that grandmother taught me to use and I slept outside in the fresh air." Eight days later he felt perfectly well and walked 40 miles to a meeting in town.

I saw a man coming into Vilcabamba with an oxygen tank on his back. He couldn't walk more than a few feet without taking a swig of oxygen. After a few days there—no more oxygen. It's hard to believe that such a thing could actually happen.

There are two rivers, one that actually comes from a volcano that is 5 or 6 miles away. When people take a bath in the river they feel so rejuvenated they could tear the shingles off the roof! I wonder if it is sulphured water or just what is there. I wondered all through my travels what causes this long life, this good health.

There is a special tree that grows in Vilcabamba called the Wilcox Tree. It doesn't grow anyplace else. It has a non-magnetic wood. The tree grows at a certain altitude, a certain climate. They don't have any snow there, any change in seasons;

it's practically the same all year round. Not only that, it is right on top of the equator. Maybe there is no pull to the south or north pole. I wondered if magnetic currents had anything to do with it. As we got up to the northern part of the country and even the southern part, there was a magnetic pull from the north and south poles. A lot of people may say this is foolishness, but I never realized this until I turned on the spigot in the wash basin. The water will always drain out to the right. But when you go down to New Zealand and turn on the water the water always goes to the left. When you look at the vines growing in this country you'll notice they always grow to the right of a pole. In New Zealand, they always grow around to the left. When you have an oil well above the equator, it will always blow towards the north pole, but down in South America, it blows towards the south pole.

When a railroad track above the equator going from east to west or west to east needs repair, it is always the north track they have to fix. The pull on that train is so great it wears out that north track. Of course, south of the equator, it is always the south track that needs repairing. Nature has many ways that we don't know very much about yet, and I'm going to give you some of these Keys that I have discovered.

I visited the University of Loja, and they told me that many people in this town had heart troubles and would go to Vilcabamba only 60 miles away to cure their troubles. Foods, habits or diets were not changed and I wondered if there was a magnetic influence in the river running through Vilcabamba where people took baths that rejuvenated them to an amazing degree.

I saw many people going to this city and their heart troubles were relieved almost immediately. I met Mr. Carpio there who was 129 years of age. He told me he has never needed the assistance of a doctor. We found a 90 year old man working as many as 10 hours a day at his craft of furniture making. We met another man. Mr. Toledo, who was 132 years of age. When he was 110 he had pneumonia, but he cured himself with herbs from the field. He claimed he recuperated with fresh air and herb teas, and then 10 days later he walked 40 miles to a meeting.

When you ask these men about their diet, they say they only eat what grows in this valley. It was a good variety of fruits and vegetables, sugar cane, corn, cereal, eggs, chickens, but very little meat.

The altitude of Vilcabamba compared to the altitude found where the elderly men lived in central Europe. They may find one of these days that there are radioactive properties which have a rejuvenating effect. Without going into this in depth, we found that those who regained their health there bragged how their sexual activity had been returned and restored. They talked about how much stronger they felt, how much their digestion had improved; and yet again there were on no special program of eating.

There is one thing we know for sure: they had black soil, lots of sunshine, the right altitude and the proper amount of ultraviolet. This valley is well named "the Sacred Valley." Many doctors have gone down to investigate this community and found that what they expected was true: these people lived a long, healthy and productive life even in old age.

We recognize that circulation and exercise are very closely related. It was in New Zealand that we came in contact with the Auckland Joggers Club; and it was here that we met Arthur Lydiard who was the champion jogger because of the work he has started in many different countries with his program. He went into this work in a very scientific manner, and coached many a person in the Olympic games and to athletic records. Like many coaches he agrees that jogging is not only fun, but it can help one live longer because it slows down the heart beat. A regular jogger can save up to 43,000 heart beats per day.

In Australia, we could see some of the inheritence key coming out in many of the people. It was reflected in their pioneering spirit by taking hold of a country that needed a lot of work. There is much drought there, and they are overcoming it by building canals, flumes, and digging for wells in the desert where many people thought there was no water to be had. In Australia they participate in sports probably more than any other place in the world. They have many different kinds of climate that are favorable in outdoor exercises. The aborigines, a stone-age people considered by anthropologists to be the most archaic civilization on the earth, possibly evolved from the Neanderthal man 300,000 years ago. They have interested scientists because of their dependence upon the natural environment without the use of cultivation or herding. They have a very mystical tie with nature and they use specific plants, animals and natural objects in their foods. They are part of their family relations; it is part of their social order and some of them are never eaten or harmed.

We find that they live very close to the soil, building their houses or huts from what they can in their environment.

They never knew any sickness until it was brought to them by people from other continents. Australia is certainly a country of contrasts where many of the Keys are found but not enough of them to produce the long life as well as a good and healthy one.

It was in Japan that I saw the effect of the sea world foods upon a person: how it affected what is probably the greatest gland in the body, the thyroid, to create a proper metabolic balance in the body. It is something to see how the glandular system is affected by the thyroid and controlled by the use of the iodine the Japanese people have so much of in their seaweed and sea fish. They have soups and even candy made of products from the sea; altogether, they make over 500 different dishes from sea products.

One of the things I discovered while I was there is that you don't find any goiter in all of Japan. However, if you go to Switzerland, high in the mountains, they all lack iodine; and many of the people have goiter, showing the effects of food upon the body.

Recently in Tokyo, an experiment was conducted to curb smog. Auto traffic was banned in four of Tokyo's busiest shopping and amusement centers for only one day. The four districts participating in the one-day test revealed that smog had been reduced to one-half. This certainly is an excellent example of group consciousness creating an impetus for good.

It was this group consciousness that you could see develop amongst those who were living the longest life. They were community minded, one for all and all for one. When one person needed a barn, they all helped to build it. If someone had a problem with their water system they all helped to rebuild or to make a new one, whatever was necessary. When you see these people work who live the long life and are the healthiest, it is clear that they recognize they cannot live by themselves, that they need one another, and that no one is an island.

City life has become a subject of great concern to the scientists and to the nature-minded person. A great example was brought out in Singapore. We found there that when old buildings were torn out, the rebuilding program must include well-planned parks with plenty of greenery. It was also brought out in New Zealand that the cities today should take more into account in their planning on how they can have more trees and greenery growing there because of the lack of ozone that the trees produce.

In Hong Kong you could see the people preparing their bodies before going to work by doing the exercises of Tai Chi. These compare a good deal to the slow, deliberate yoga exercises as demonstrated in India. Tai Chi gives poise and a definite tempo that the body can live with. It involves 108 phases of body motion based on animal movement. Tai Chi stresses slow breathing; a balanced, relaxed posture; and an absolute calmness of mind. The Chinese believe that Tai Chi develops inner poise and thereby prolongs the state of youth. Tai Chi is becoming quite popular, and we see it being taught in parks in this country.

We were very interested in the philosophy and the past history of the Chinese people. They had developed that positive and negative philosophy of yin and yang. They had been using acupuncture that had developed 2,000 years before Christ, and people are just discovering it now and finding out how wonderful it really is. China had much to give to us and probably will have much more in the years to come.

In taking out the fine things in all of our travels we were looking for the things that could affect humanity in the greatest way possible from a health and long life standpoint; and we saw that the treatment of mankind was very necessary in both gaining and maintaining health, and in preventing disease.

For example, in China the doctor of the past would claim that he would have to have a patient over a period of at least six months so he could get to know his family, his inheritance, his work, his marriage, and how well he gets along with other people. After this six month period, then the doctor claimed he could help you.

It was a great moment when I came upon the history of Li Ching Yun. He truly was a great example when we think that he lived to the age of 256. He outlived 23 wives. But one of the great Keys I consider to be most important of all was expressed by him just before he died when he was asked to what he attributed his long life, and he replied, "Inward Calm." I personally believe this is one of the greatest sermons I have ever heard, and certainly is badly needed in civilization today.

Li Chung Yun, of Kaihsien, in the Province of Szechwan, China, was born in 1677 and died in 1933 at the age of 256 years. A professor in the Minkuo University claims to have found records showing that Li was born in 1677, and that on his 150th birthday, in 1827, he was congratulated by the Chinese government. Fifty years later, in 1877, he was sent another official congratulation on his 200th birthday. Fifty years later, at the age of 250 years, he lectured before several thousand university students for many hours at a time on the art of living long. Men who are old today declare that their great grandfathers, as boys, knew Li as a grown man. He had 24 successive wives and eleven generations of descendants.

Early in life, Li developed an interest in herbs, and especially in ginseng, and for the greater part of his long life he wandered round collecting herbs and selling them. He was especially interested in collecting the best specimens of wild ginseng, and for two centuries he partook of ginseng tea four times daily.

NEWSPAPER ARTICLES ON LI-CHING-YUN

London Times—May 8, 1933 Column G (Title of Column: "Telegrams in Brief")

A telegram from Chungking in the province of Szechwan, CHINA, states that LI-CHING-YUN, reputed to be the oldest man in China and presumably in the world, has died at Kiah-Sien, at the alleged age of 256.—Reuters

New York Times, Saturday, May 6, 1933; page 13, Col. 4:

LI-CHING-YUN-DEAD;
GAVE HIS AGE AS 197

'Keep quiet Heart, Sit Like a
Tortoise, Sleep Like a Dog'
His advice for Long Life.

INQUIRY PUT AGE AT 256

Reported to have buried 23 wives
and had 180 Descendants—Sold
Herbs for First 100 Years.

PEIPING, May 5 (AP) Li-Ching-Yun, a resident of Kaihsien, in the Province of Szechwan, who contended that he was one of the world's oldest men and said he was born in 1736—which would make him 197 years old—died today.

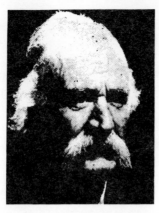

A Chinese dispatch from Chungking telling of Mr. Li's death said he attributed his longevity to peace of mind and that it was his belief that every one could live at least a century by attaining inward calm.

Compared with estimates of Li-Ching-Yun's age in previous reports from China the above dispatch is conservative. In 1930 it was said Professor Wu-Chung-Chien, Dean of the Department of Education in Minkuo University, had found records showing Li was born in 1677 and that the Imperial Chinese Government congratulated him on his 150th and 200th birthdays.

A correspondent of the NEW YORK TIMES wrote in 1928 that many of the oldest men in Li's neighborhood asserted their grandfathers knew him as boys and that he was then a grown man.

According to generally accepted tales told in his province, Li was able to read and write as a child, and by his tenth birthday had traveled in Kansu, Shansi, Tibet, Annam, Siam and Manchuria gathering herbs. For the first hundred years he continued at this occupation. Then he switched to selling herbs gathered by others.

Wu-Pei-Fu, the war lord, took Li into his house to learn the secret of living to 250. Another pupil said Li told him to "keep a quiet heart, sit like a tortoise, walk sprightly like a pigeon, and sleep like a dog."

According to one version of Li's married life he had buried 23 wives and was living with his 24th, a woman of 60. Another account, which in 1928 credited him with 180 living descendants, comprising 11 generations, recorded only 14 marriages. This second authority said his eyesight was good; also that the finger nails of his right hand were very long, and "long" for a

Chinese might mean longer than any finger nails ever dreamed of in the United States.

One statement of the TIMES correspondent which probably caused skeptical readers to believe Li was born more recently than 1677, was that "many who have seen him recently declare that his facial appearance is no different from that of persons two centuries his junior."

(Note: The N.Y. Times article of May 8, 1933 merely repeats his age and makes some comic observations of world events he would have witnessed if he actually were 197 when he died.)

I became acquainted with the Indian runners in New Mexico and Arizona when we heard about the different runners throughout the world. In years past they had runners carrying the seafoods inland to people who had goiters and found that this was their medicine. They developed the ability of these runners. The Olympics games are always preceded by the marathon runner who demonstrates his stamina by running for some 26 miles. Many people do not realize that back in the Grecian days when they had these marathon runners, the prize for the man who won was a stalk of celery.

I had a good friend, Mr. Larry Lewis, who was 106 years of age. He certainly was a grand example of a man who had strength and endurance. He was a waiter at the St. Francis Hotel in San Francisco when he was 106 years old. He ran six miles every morning before breakfast, and he said his formula for long life was to keep the body and mind active. "Work never hurt anybody, only worry, and so I work." He believed in simple foods, and he doesn't smoke or drink. He said some people hate their jobs and can't wait for retirement, but he thinks this is a mistake because nobody should retire at any age. Larry said, "Work keeps the brain active and gives a person a reason for living." He feels that by the time people reach 65 they are just beginning to put to use the things they have learned. Larry also claimed that if you wanted to have good health you had to drink lots of water.

In traveling around the world, of course I wanted to know where the oldest people were here in the U.S. In seeking out the oldest person, I found Charlie Smith in the picturesque town of Bartow, Florida, tucked away in the interior of the state. He is the oldest living American, 133 years of age, and was born in Liberia, Africa in 1842. Charlie recalls that when he was 12 years old a big boat docked and a white man enticed him and many others to come aboard ship. When they got them aboard, the slave ship set sail. He was sold as a slave to a Capt. Charlie Smith, a wealthy Texas land owner who gave Charlie his name. When asked about his diet he said he ate most anything, "but I don't eat much cooked ration and I don't have no certain time to eat." He told me he eats only when hungry.

When discussing diet with him, he really astounded me when he told me he had been living primarily on crackers and sardines. Maybe there is something in the sardine that we should investigate. It has kept this man going well in his elderly years. Possibly the sardines should be considered a whole food, having the calcium, silicon, sodium, phosphorous and various other elements that we need for the body to use in a well balanced way.

Charlie is probably the oldest man on Social Security in the United States, and he said that his main rule for long life is his faith in God. He told me that another thing that keeps him feeling good is singing. One of the things he mentions that keeps him in good health is going to bed early. When you look at some of the Keys for this elderly man, you can see that he has led quite a life that included horseback riding, living out on the plains and breaking horses. He also rode with Billy the Kid in his younger years, though he claimed he never shot anybody. He was one who was involved in the heavy physical exercise that was found in the West and on the Texas plains.

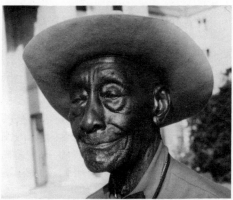

Charlie Smith, 133-years-old, is the United States oldest citizen.

Chapter 6

Lessons of the Aged

My search for longevity continued throughout Western Europe and the Balkan countries, leading me finally to Turkey, long known for its history of strong and healthy people.

For centuries, the world viewed Turkey as both a bridge and a barrier: a bridge, because its trade-routes served as a crossroad between Europe, Asia and Africa; and a barrier, because its boundaries limited the expansion of numerous neighboring countries. Consequently, many wars have been waged over this strategically located country.

For six centuries, from twelve hundred and ninety to nineteen hundred and twenty two, Turkey was without peace. As a result it became a melting pot of races, and the intermingling of many blood strains resulted.

In Eastern Turkey, near the Armenian border, is a peninsula of land lying between the Black and Caspian Seas, which connects Turkey with Iran and Russia, known as the Caucasus.

This territory has been called a "Garden of Eden" because of its mild climate and rich soil. Grapes grow in this part of the world, and you find wherever people live a long life grapes are growing. There is a long growing season for grapes and vegetables. There have also been more wars where these old people are living than anywhere else. There have been 200 wars in the last 1,000 years in this one particular place. This is what people are fighting for: for land that produces the right kind of food.

History reports that soldiers from every invading army from the Assyrians to the Crusaders to the Turks settled in the fertile valleys of the Caucasus mountain regions. It was here that investigators thought they had located the perfect type of white race which is still called Caucasian.

I visited with two elderly men working in the fields. Cafer is 100 years old and Omar is 99. Both are devout Moslems. They rise early, and retire early. Their diet consists of yogurt, fruits, vegetables, seeds, nuts, and grains. Meat is served about twice a week.

As we traveled the mountainous country south of Trabazon we passed a spry and obviously very strong lady carrying a heavy load. Strength is one of these people's outstanding characteristics.

In Turkey, I observed that the unschooled peasants were most often the longest living people. Walking on roads, working in fields which are built on mountainous terrain has developed a stamina and vitality in these Turks that lasts a lifetime.

In the cities, as well as in the rural areas, I was most impressed with the great strength displayed by the elderly. I met a man 82 years old, carrying a piano! And I was amazed to learn that the wrestling champion of Turkey was 75 years old.

The Turks claim that the secret to their robust health is the sesame seed. This may well be, for wherever I found the strongest elderly people, I noticed that a large percentage of their diet consisted of foods rich in potassium, which is a muscle building element in the body. They also eat a lot of seeds from melons and squash. Their olives are preserved in sea salt, and chestnuts are a regular part of their diet.

The Turks eat no white bread, for the government requires a minimum of 6 percent bran in all bread. And in Turkey, a goat is man's best friend. Even in their candy, they use sesame seed mixed with a concentrated grape juice.

About 20 miles outside Trabazon, I met a gentleman of 108 years of age. I also met a 110-year-old lady who never had any ailments. She didn't even know what the word "arthritis" meant.

In Erzurum, we arranged to meet a 132-year-old man who was brought to town from his mountain home. But, he was not very cooperative. It seems that a local reporter had written erroneously that he was looking for a very young wife. He was one of the very few men we saw with a bent-over condition.

My inspiration to visit these people came from studying Alexander the Great and his travels. As I traced his course I found that his strongest men came from this area which is now Turkey. It was, however, expanded at that time and it is now considered part of Russia.

My efforts were concentrated in this area because I felt there were more people past the century mark, still working and possessing this great strength.

The following photographic examples illustrate the physical characteristics of these people. These are the calcium people; angular and bony. Their digestive systems were excellent; their sexual systems strong; and they were muscular. We found them living in the mountains, out of the cities.

These people were the finest warriors because of their tenacity and endurance. The type of warfare fought in the past employed this sheer physical strength. Cities were conquered by the perseverance of these "Terrible Turks" as they were known.

However, their family life has always been of great importance to them and the preservation of the family unit and their land were the reasons for the stalwart defense of their territory.

A main part of their diet consisted of sesame seeds, olives, garlic, sunflower seeds, vegetables, greens, clabbered milk, fruits, natural herbs.

I can truthfully say that these people had more of the World Keys than any other group of people we visited.

From Turkey, we traveled a short distance across the border, into Armenia. I found it a fascinating land, a mixture of ancient buildings, crude villages and medieval ruins which were constant reminders of Armenia's long and stormy history. Our destination was a rural area on the outskirts of Spidek, where I was told I would find some old people.

The first elderly person I interviewed was a 110-year-old woman. She told me her diet consisted mostly of clabbered milk, raw vegetables, fruits, and seeds from squash, melons, sunflowers, and sesame. She had all her mental faculties and was still leading a useful life.

A short distance away, a group of her relatives gathered in honor of our visit. Two elderly ladies put on their "Sunday best" for the occasion. My interpreter, Mr. Ghazarian, inquired about their ages. The lady replied, "I am 127, and my daughter is 85!" Their relatives reported that these women are active, alert, contented and devout.

The 127-year-old lady said she has worked all her life, and likes it. We asked her what she thought contributed to her many years and she replied, "comfrey leaf and garlic, dried, made into a soup." She also said she used rose-hip tea, which she believed kept her family free of winter complaints.

It is most interesting that for centures, garlic has been regarded with what is close to reverence by people all over the world. Even Plato noted that garlic can be used 61 ways for good health. It should also be noted that children at celebrations are given sunflower seeds, not candy!

Periodically, fairs are held to award prizes for quality produce. In an area where longevity was not unusual, I was not surprised to see so much emphasis placed upon the growing of wholesome fruits and vegetables.

The regard for quality food was evident throughout Armenia. In Erevan, I visited one of the most impressive markets I've ever seen, both outside and inside! And over the past ten years, the output of produce from this area has increased 1,000 percent!

The Armenians opened their hearts and homes to us. They truly believe in the brotherhood of man, and they proudly claim their country to be the oldest Christian state.

I wanted to go next to Azerbaijan in the Soviet Union where the oldest people in Russia are located. Although it was only a distance of 80 miles from where I was in Armenia, it necessitated my traveling back to Istanbul, then all the way to Moscow to secure permission from the Soviet authorities to visit the old people who resided in the mountain area outside of Baku.

WHAT THE LONG-LIVED PEOPLE ATE

Among the inhabitants of Dagestan, many people over 100 years of age are to be found. The records obtained by H. J. Mustafaev concerning the food of the elderly show that they used a rather large amount of albumen, amounting to about 110 grams a day in the form of boiled milk, Kefir (a fermented liquor made from milk), curdle milk, sour cream, curds, and goat cheese. They eat meat only once or twice a week and practically no fish nor fish products, while as to sugar, they eat at most two or three lumps a day. They take carbohydrates chiefly as dishes made of flour, rice, potatoes, peas, and honey. They satisfy their needs in fats by eating butter, mutton, and beef fats. They do not recognize any alcoholic drinks; they do not drink coffee; nor do they eat chocolate, cream tarts, or smoked sausage and pork.

In all parts of and among all the various peoples of Dagestan, the favorite dish is the Hinmal* containing meat and garlic!

[1]"Problems of Feeding" 1973 N$_3$, P. 46 USSR

*Large flat cakes boiled in a sieve and spiced according to taste.

It was autumn when we arrived in Russia. In the city of Moscow I was surprised to see women doing so much manual labor.

My purpose in coming to Moscow was to see government officials in the Kremlin with the hope they would grant me permission to visit the famous old people of Russia. I was also hoping to obtain certificates attesting to their age.

The Kremlin is one of the greatest remaining monuments of medieval Russian architecture. It is virtually a town of palaces, churches and government buildings, surrounded by walls 12 feet high and 40 feet thick.

My visit to the Kremlin proved most rewarding. I received the fullest co-operation from the authorities and was granted permission to conduct my research on Russia's oldest living people.

While at the Kremlin, I visited the region of the central squares, the most famous of which is Red Square, the site of Lenin's Tomb.

Here in the central squares are located the main governmental buildings, the more important theaters and hotels, and the main shopping district.

We visited the largest department store in the world. If I were to attempt to describe its size, I'm afraid I would be accused of gross exaggeration.

The famous church where Count Leo Tolstoy was married held a particular interest for me, because I have always been an admirer of his literary achievements.

With my mission accomplished I headed back to our hotel, which incidentally had 6,000 rooms.

The next morning we took off for Baku, the capital city of the Azerbaijan Socialist Soviet Republic. One of our memorable experiences in this city was an exciting cable car ride, which gave us a thrilling view of this vast metropolis.

The chief product of Baku is petroleum, which at one time caused heavy pollution; but now the air is clear due to a modern technique of trapping the oil soot. The entire process is vacuum sealed.

I found the inhabitants of Baku to be very health-minded. One indication of this was the daily calisthenic program conducted in the parks. Throughout this area, an estimated 150,000 people turn out each morning to exercise.

The calisthenics impressed me as having some of the free-flowing movements of ballet. The graceful, rhythmical stretch of muscles seems to be the keynote of each exercise. All of these exercises were done with music.

Finally, I was on my way to meet the second oldest living person in the world, Mr. Shirin Gasanov, 153 years of age. The man was absolutely amazing. He had the skin texture, vitality, and carriage of a youthful man.

The Russian authorities arranged to have him brought to meet me for a television interview, and during this interview Mr. Gasanov revealed his health secrets to our interpreter.

Mr. Gasanov says he enjoys life. He does not drink or smoke. He is at peace with the world!

We could see this was a vigorous man, although he told us he had developed pneumonia at the age of 148 and refused to take medicine from the doctors because he preferred the fresh air and herbs as treatment.

According to his passport, this man was born in 1817; yet he was out at 6 a.m. every morning working with the other farmers. Continuing with his daily work, is of course, one of the main Keys to his long life. Active and alert, he rode a horse until the age of 148 when the doctors wanted him to stop.

The Russians have assigned special doctors to these old people. Dr. Kiamal Mirzoev, who periodically examined Mr. Gasanov, reports that his health is superior to that of a normal, middle-aged person. He reports that Gasanov's blood pressure is 130, over 80, and he has a strong pulse of 75 beats per minute.

When I inquired about his eating habits, he told us that during the last six years he ate according to a special diet. He said, "I eat very little in the evening and have my last meal at 6 o'clock. After 6 o'clock, I do not eat." He partakes of foods sparingly, not overeating. Milk products are a large part of his diet, including sour cream, sour milk and matsoni. Vegetables and fruits are used as well as some boiled meat. Years ago he was a vegetarian, and now he does eat meat, but very seldom. Both cooked and fresh foods are used and he eats kasha (buckwheat groats) with milk. Although herbs from the field may be used to treat ailments, he drinks very little, but does drink a lot of water.

Mr. Gasanov told us he usually stays in his own village and rarely travels. Most of the people, about 70% of the population in his village, are his own relatives!

At the age of 15 he married for the first time. His third wife had 12 children and he now has many, many grandchildren.

The age of his youngest child is 60; he was 93 when that child was born and his wife was 73. The doctor says that in

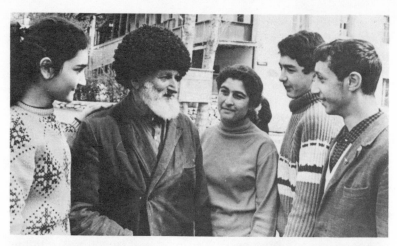

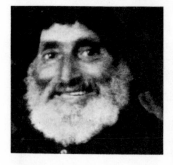

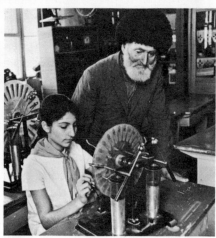

Shirin Gasanov of Russia at 153 years of age.

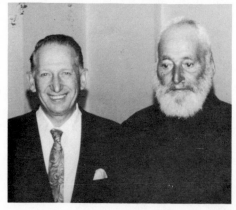

Dr. Jensen and Mr. Gasanov.

their region there are 12 men who were fathers after the age of 90.

In his youth Gasanov was a poor man, living in the mountains as a shepherd. There was no special menu, no special food, as he tells us: "I was a very poor man. You were asking about my menu, what time did I eat, what did I eat; but I tell you this, sometimes I didn't eat, not even bread. Sometimes I drank water from the rivers, no menu, no special foods." He did not rest much when he was younger, as he was from a poor family and was always working. He had to work in order to eat. Of course, this activity through most of his life was an important Key to his longevity, but he did say in recent years his life has been easier.

Longevity is not a stranger to this region, or to his family, for his mother died at the age of 90 and his father died at the age of 100 years. One sister lived until 140, and several other relatives lived until the ages of 100 and 110. He mentioned that one of his grandchildren died at the age of 97, and he has over 100 grandchildren and great-grandchildren.

Gasanov is a religious man and does pray, he says. He neither drinks nor smokes. We inquired of his philosophy, Was he a happy man? Did he like music? He replied, "I myself like music very well because I am from the place where the music belonged to everybody. There are many musicians from Azerbaijan and we are very famous for our music."

We also learned that   Gasanov was a counselor in his village. He is respected as a wise man, and the people come to him for advice.

In parting, he leaned toward me and said, "If you really want to live a long life, control your temper, help other people, and love everybody."

I shall carry with me always the image of this unusual man, beautiful in spirit, mind and body.

RUSSIAN CERTIFICATE: This is to inform you that Shirin Gasanogly Gasanov, a native of the Chereken Village of the Dzhebrailskiy district, Azerbaijan, SSR, is of Azerbaijanian nationality, a farmer, and according to the entries in the collective Farm Register and his passport, was born 1, July, 1817. (Director of the Office of Notaries and Records of Vital Statistics at the Ministry of Justice, Azerbaijan, SSR.)

Next, we headed for the Talysh mountains where the oldest man in the world lives. On the way, I visited with quite a number of elderly people.

We met a spry old gentlemen of 92 years of age. He ate a

variety of simple foods, such as grains, tomatoes, cucumbers, green onions, mutton, beef, fruits, berries, and vegetables such as peas, cabbage, turnips and peppers.

The elderly people eat many kinds of seeds from squash, melons, sunflower and sesame; and about 60% of their vegetables are eaten raw.

Like their mates, the elderly women maintained excellent posture and seemed to possess boundless energy. One key that was certainly common to all of the old people was their routine of working from sunup to sunset.

We met a gentleman of 100 years of age, and like his fellow countrymen, he uses over 200 varieties of wild plants and herbs, which he eats both cooked and raw.

Certainly a candidate for the select circle of oldest living humans in the world is Mr. Frazal, 142 years of age. Like the rest of the elderly, he will never retire. He says that work is one of the keys to health and that when he works he does only what he is capable of doing. He makes no demands on himself that he cannot meet. With his age, his status in the community increases. All of the people we saw of advanced age, with only a few exceptions, were married.

I think this is significant in view of the gerontologists who say that a married state extends longevity. I was told that another key to their long life was the traditional habit of men not marrying before the age of 30 in order to preserve their sexual energies.

In the Talysh mountains we found a colony of old people living a peaceful life in an alpine setting.

All paid homage to these venerable old gentlemen, who told me that they go to bed at the same time each night, and they sleep in the fresh air for about 8 months of the year. Only in winter do they sleep in rooms.

"Kindness," these old gentlemen told me, "is a quality which decorates a person better than precious stones. The malicious do not live long."

How refreshing to see age revered, rather than considered a burden on society.

Shirali Mislimov, at 168 years of age, was the oldest living person in the world. Although the Soviet government did not allow him to be interviewed, I was fortunate in getting these pictures of him.

Riding horseback was his favorite pastime, except when he had the opportunity to talk to young people.

Shirali was a sheepherder, as were most of these elderly

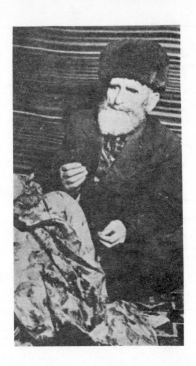

Shirali Mislimov's relatives number 220. He came to Baku only three times in his life on business and was never sick a day in his life. His pulse 70-72 and blood pressure 125/75. This is usual for a person at the ages between 30 to 40 years.

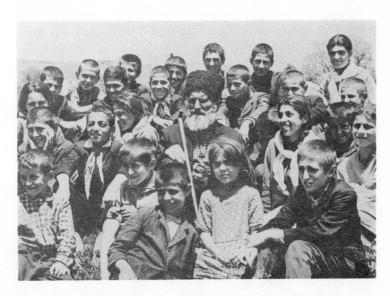

people. Apparently, walking over the mountainous terrain developed hard leg muscles which are responsible for the excellent muscle tone and cardiovascular fitness of these old people.

They were happy and satisfied with what they had. They never rushed anywhere and they told me they were not in a hurry to die.

All of them were family people, which indicates that family life favors good health.

Their diet remained the same throughout their lives. Nuts and berries are an important staple in their diet. Their food is naturally grown without commercial fertilizers or sprays.

I found many elderly couples who had been married eighty, ninety, and even a hundred years. It seemed that the women with the most children, lived the longest.

Matsoni, is a complete protein, easy to digest, and a whole food.

A popular way of eating clabbered milk, among the elders, is to mix it with honey, and eat it with bread. Their bread is stone-ground and very coarse.

They pick their own herbs from the fields which they grind and make into teas. Camomile and rose hips are favorite teas. They drink herb teas frequently throughout the day, and regard it as a natural remedy.

Another contributing factor to their good health, is their pure mountain water.

I wrote a letter to Mr. Mislimov and we include a copy of this letter as sent to him. You will note in the reply that he did not answer the questions one by one but incorporated them in his letter.

I think he sums up most of the Keys that help give us the long life and good health.

I do consider this letter from him to be one of the nicest letters I have ever received in my life.

October 5, 1972
Mr. Shirali Mislimov
Dear Mr. Mislimov:

I am a doctor who has a very great interest in the subject of longevity.

I have been to Russia twice in the last few years, and I wanted to meet you, but it did not prove to be convenient.

I did meet Mr. Gasanov while in Baku and found that to be a great pleasure and honor.

I have a few questions I would like to ask you for my research, and would appreciate it if you could give me some answers on them. Do you feel that there are any special foods that help you to feel healthy and active?

What are your favorite foods?

What do you eat in the winter when the weather is very cold?

Do you believe in fasting?

What is your daily routine and your typical diet for the day?

Do you believe in three meals a day?

Do you drink much milk? Or, is the milk in the form of a clabber?

Do you use much honey?

How many times a week do you eat meat?

At what altitude do you live?

How much schooling have you had?

Have you been getting thinner as you grow older?

I have always thought that the muscles in the legs were very important for good circulation of blood throughout the body. Do you walk a lot?

What time do you go to bed and what time do you rise in the morning?

Has your physical activity been diminishing the last 10-20 years?

Have you any stiffness in any of the joints?

What rules do you have for living so long?

What mental philosophy would you give a young man like me at the age of 65 to follow?

How many children have you?

How many times have you been married?

Are you married now?

One of these days we expect to be in the U.S.S.R. again, and would like to have the opportunity of seeing you. I would appreciate receiving a photograph of you that you have signed.

I want to wish you much happiness and a wonderful life ahead.

Sincerely yours,
Dr. Bernard Jensen

Dear Dr. Jensen:

Many thanks for your kind letter of October 5, 1972. I wish to answer you as follows:

As to your first question, I want to tell you that I do not use any special food at all. I eat ordinary food, just as all other mountaineers do.

Best of all, I prefer our national dish—pilau, which consists of rice boiled in milk, with butter.

In winter when the cold weather begins, I eat milk-gruel, honey, cheese, chicken broth, boiled fruit and especially soup prepared with sour milk (matsoni).

Yes, I believe in fasting. I eat very little mutton and salty dishes. I have hardly ever observed any diet. I drink milk when I feel like it; I drink it every day and eat whenever I feel hungry. I have never kept to any fixed time for meals. When I feel hungry I mostly drink clabber-milk and eat cottage cheese (milk-curd). I seldom have honey—once or twice a week, and as to meat, I eat minced beef in the form of cutlets or rolled in cabbage leaves, twice a week.

I live at an altitude of 1,700 meters above the sea-level in a mountainous village surrounded by forests.

I have never attended school as, at those distant years when I was small, there were no schools in Caucasian villages.

As I grew older I did not get much thinner as even in my young days my body-frame was about the same as it is now.

I am used to taking walks for about one kilometer a day. My legs do not ache as walking is a habit of mine.

You are quite right when you consider that not only the muscles of the legs, but also of the arms and other muscles are very important for good circulation of the blood throughout the body; and that is why I feel exceptionally well after my walks or any other physical exercise.

I usually get up early in the morning and go to bed at about 10 o'clock at night. I do not like to sleep during the day and in the day-time I never feel sleepy.

As I grow older I feel that my physical activity is giving way. For instance, I can no more lift weights of from 20 to 25 kilograms as I used to ten years ago.

I have no stiffness in my joints and I am as agile as I have always been all my life.

It has never occurred to me before to observe and I have never observed any special rules to attain old age. A quiet family life, mountain climate and the happy life of my descendants—that is what accounts for my long life.

My advice is as follows: Be always noble and generous, take care of other peoples' and of your own health. Take more walks and be less nervous.

I was married three times. During our joint life we had 23 children, of which only two remain. My third wife Khatoon is 107 years old. She also feels quite well and looks after me.

Much esteem, Dr. Bernard Jensen! Warm thanks for your kind attention and good wishes towards me. I also wish you every success in your honorable work, and much happiness in your family life. I wish you to live as long as I.

I'm sending you my autograph.

Yours respectfully,
Shirali Mislimov

February 15, 1973

BULGARIA

When traveling to Bulgaria I realized that I was in a country where it has been claimed that there are more people over the age of 100 years of age, according to their population, than any other country in the world. Of course, I wanted to know why. What kind of people were they? They live a peasant life, a hard life, one that builds a good body.

What were they living on? We find that they are famous for their clabbered milk, their Bulgarian buttermilk, the greatest food to feed the friendly bacteria in the large intestinal tract. It is the bacteria that keeps the colon sweet and clean and active. Professor Metchnikoff claimed that keeping the bowel clean and having plenty of the friendly bacteria is very important. There are many experiments that we had worked out with patients who had bowel disturbances and colon problems, and we found this friendly bacteria was important in establishing the proper intestinal flora.

The Trappist Monks in Canada have continued the culture of the Bulgarian bacteria so it would not die. The health food stores are blessed with this food, but it is because the Trappist Monks have kept this culture alive. The Monks are still making cheese and cultures for the industry throughout the U.S. and Canada.

I am convinced that these people live at a certain altitude where the milk develops a bacteria because of the altitude and climate. The milk comes from animals that are fed on grasses and greens that grow at a certain altitude to develop this bacteria best.

If the average person took an acidophilus culture a couple of months, two or three times a year, it would be to their advantage and would add to their health and life span.

Elimination and digestion are very important, and these people had this particular Key developed to a marked degree.

Los Angeles Herald-Examiner, Wednesday, February 12, 1975

Russ Passes 140th Year

MOSCOW (AP) — Mejid Agayev, oldest citizen in an Azerbaijan village that numbers among its inhabitants 54 people over 100, recently celebrated his 140th birthday, Tass reported Tuesday.

The mountainous village of Tikyaband in the southern Soviet republic is described as "a village of centenarians," Tass said. But it is not uncommon for residents of the mountains in Azerbaijan and Georgia to reach 100 years.

The Soviet news agency did not say if Agayev was the oldest man in the village. It said he is alert and continues his favorite occupation, wood carving.

Shirali Mislimov, an Azerbaijani farmer claimed to be the oldest man in the world, died in 1973 at the age of 168, Soviet officials said.

Azerbaijan ranks 1st in the world in the number of long life people. They have 84 people of 100 years of age or older for every 100,000 in the Republic.

90

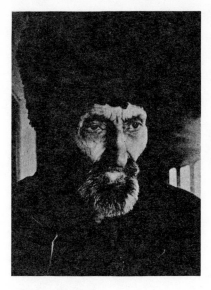

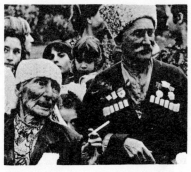

KHFAR TARKUKOVNA LASURIA:
140 years of age

Has worked all her life in tea plantations and citrus orchards.
Has never been ill or visited a doctor.
Sociable and hospitable.
Has a good sense of humor.
Smokes and drinks.
Pictured with her son who is a centernarian.

BALAKISKY:
137 years of age.

When he passed away in 1969 his wife, Anina, 120 years of age, was still living.
He was a farmer all of his life and a hard worker.
Diet mostly was: sour milk, chicken, fish, honey, meat, vegetables, homemade bread, quinces.
Had his own garden.
Never sick—died suddenly in one week's time.
Son was 65.

MEDZHID AGAEV:
134 years of age.

In the village of Tikyaband is the oldest shepherd in the world.
He covers 6 to 7 miles every-day walking along mountain paths.
His diet consists of dairy products, honey, sheep-milk cheese and greens.
He eats 4 small meals a day.
His favorite beverage is water.
He has never tasted liquor.

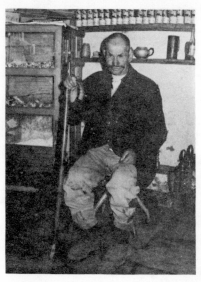

ISKENDER KARAKAS:
128 years of age.

Born in Caucasus [according
to 65-year-old son, he is over
128].
Came to Turkey in 1910.
Married first at 17; married 6
times since.
Robust and vigorous.
Farmer and shepherd in
youth; later a porter.
Has had a difficult and hard
life.
Hasn't been examined or taken
any pills.
Cannot see clearly or hear
perfectly.
Fasts in Ramazan but doesn't
worship.
Started smoking after 50.
Smokes 20-25 a day.
Eats 3 lbs. of meat weekly.
Uses milk, yogurt, bread and
butter.
Doesn't drink coffee or tea.

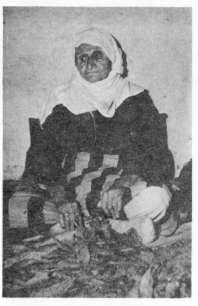

SEHER AYSE AYDIN:
112 years of age.

Joyous and happy.
Married at 16.
Likes all kinds of foods,
especially milk, yogurt, bread
and meat [3 lbs. a month].
Hears and sees poorly.
Knows nothing about pills.
When young, worked in
fields. Has had a hard life.
Very religious. Worships 5
times daily and fasts during
Ramadan.
For breakfast usually has
bread, milk, butter, jam and
sometimes tea.

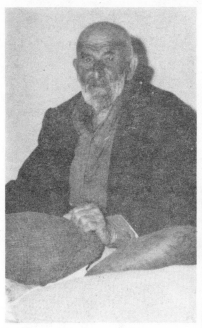

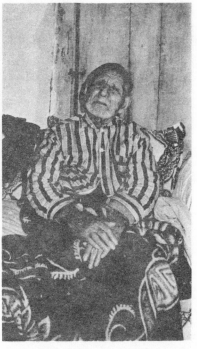

OSMAN UZUN:
110 years of age.

Born in village near Trabzon.
Still lives there.
Eats vegetables, milk, yogurt,
butter, maize bread, some
fruits, little meat, no fish or
jam.
Eats 4 or 5 times daily, but not
great quantities.
Married twice—first at age 20
and then again at 62.
Has 5 sons and 1 daughter.
Youngest son is 42, oldest is
80. All children still alive.
Religious man. Worships 5
times daily, fasts in Ramadan.
Smokes 15 cigarettes daily,
doesn't drink.
Hears well, sees poorly,
speaks slowly.
Joyous, robust, vigorous.
Walks well.

HACI HAYDAR PASA:
117 years of age.

Born near Trabzon and moved
there in 1960.
During youth worked in
fields. Sold eggs and tinplate
in Trabzon.
Very religious. Cried when
told religious stories.
Made pilgrimage 5 years ago.
Sad because he can't worship
for 10 days due to ill health.
Eats all kinds of food, drinks
little milk, much tea.
Never smoked and doesn't
drink. Eats 3 times daily.
Speaks slowly, hears poorly,
although he did hear well
before his illness.

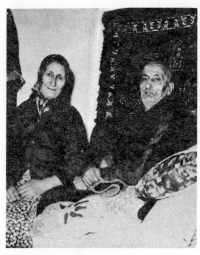

CAFER BAYKAM:
115 years of age.

In bed at home in Erzurum.
Not ill, just likes being in bed.
Sons claim he is 120.
Born in Caucasus, came to
Turkey in 1903.
First married at 40. Wife died
1 year later. Married again
at 43.
Youngest child is 13 years old.
Wants to marry again. Says if
he could find a beautiful girl,
15-16 years old, he
could live longer.
Feels men should not marry
before 35.
Traveled much when younger
as his job was trade.
Sees well, hears poorly, never
has been examined.
Hasn't worshipped since 1968
due to hemorrhoids.
Fasts in Ramadan.
Mother died at 135. Doesn't
know about father.
Smokes.
Eats yogurt, butter, bread,
mutton [2 lbs. weekly], little
fruit. Drinks milk daily.

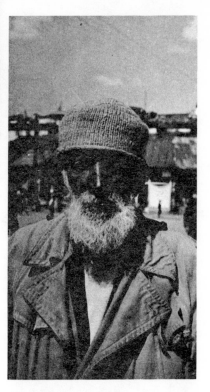

HASAN HUSNU KOL:
126 years of age.

Born in Erivan, Russia in
1844. Came to Turkey when
he was 13.
Has 90-year-old wife, still
living. Has 6 sons.
Eats milk, yogurt, bread,
apples and fish.
Does not drink tea or coffee.
Never smoked.
Still works as a shepherd.
Very poor man.
Worships and fasts in
Ramadan. Hasn't made
pilgrimage because so poor.
After taking his picture, was
given money and was very
glad. Sees well, hears poorly.

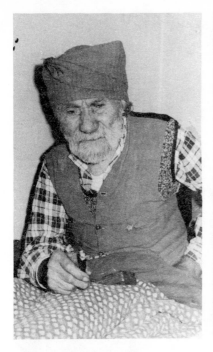

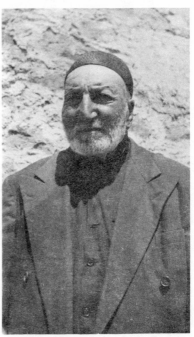

HILAL CAGISLAR:
120 years of age.

NESIM ATES:
114 years of age.

Born in Caucasia, 1850.
Came to Turkey when 15.
Mother died at 110.
A farmer, but hasn't worked
in fields for the past few years.
Was in military service for
6 years from age 68-74.
Fought in war against the
Russians.
Worships and fasts in
Ramadan. Didn't make the
pilgrimage.
Sees well, hears poorly.
Seems to be robust.
Uses milk, yogurt, butter,
bread, cheese, meat [2 lbs.
per week], some fruits.
Started drinking tea after 80.
Doesn't drink coffee.
Smokes 10 cigarettes daily.
Sleeps more than 8 hours
daily.

Born near Kars [now
U.S.S.R.].
Moved to Trabzon 45 years
ago. Worked in fields at
village near Kars.
Used to drink milk there, but
now drinks tea at Trabzon
because very poor.
Eats all kinds of foods.
Smokes 50 home-made
cigarettes daily.
Doesn't drink.
Porter in Trabzon till 95.
Then sold eggs and other
things till 112. No hard work
last 2 years.
Eats 4 times daily.
Hears well, can't see clearly,
has strong voice.
Not very religious.
Fasts only in Ramadan.

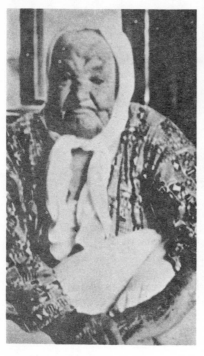

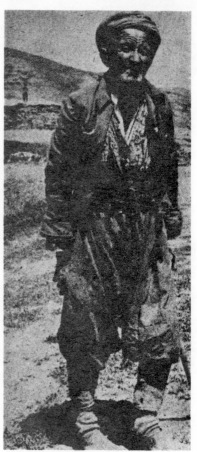

CENGIZ DEDE:
120 years of age.

HAVVA ISIKLI:
120 years of age.

Lives in Trabzon.
Worked in fields.
Eats all kinds of foods
especially milk, yogurt, meat,
cornbread and cabbage.
Eats 3 times a day.
Has never been examined.
Used to fast and worship, but
can't now.
When young, happy and
joked a lot.
Used to walk around often.

Lives in village in Turkey.
Has been widower for past 40
years. Looking for a wife to
leave his land and worldly
possessions.
Anyone interested, please
contact him.

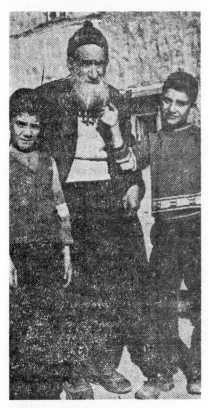

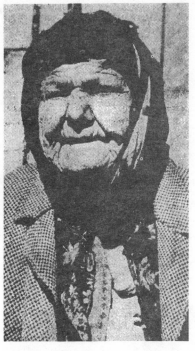

COK YASAMANIN SIMI:
119 years of age.

Works in garden like a young
man. For a long life, says eat
yogurt with garlic and drink
tea instead of water.
Served 18 years in the
military, has no other
occupation.
Works in fresh air for
2 hours daily.

HATUK NINE:
128 years of age.

Turkey's oldest lady Town
Crier. Has been the Town
Crier for the last 75 years in
the village of Resadiyie.
Strong, full voice.
Can be heard 2 blocks away.
Claims her fine health and
good voice is due to daily
breakfast of 1 quart pure
spring water mixed with lots
of lemon juice and nothing
else.

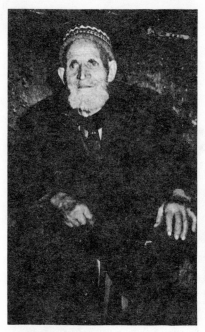

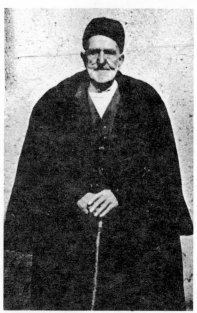

YUSUF VELIOGLU:
102 years of age.

Born in Erzurum.
Mother died at 107.
Married twice. Has 3 sons,
1 daughter.
Sons wealthy, but he lives
alone in small house as he
does not want to live
with them.
After military service became
farmer and shepherd.
Has 10 cows.
Very religious man.
Made pilgrimage 4 times.
Sees and hears well, has
strong voice.
Robust and vigorous.
Only taken 5 aspirin in
entire life.
Eats yogurt, milk, cheese,
bread, onions, meat [6 lbs.
a week]. Has 5 cups of tea
a day.
Happy and joyous.

HACI MIRZA AGA:
113 years of age.

Lives near Tebriz.
Married 3 times. Has 6 sons.
Lives with 57-year-old wife
and wants to marry again but
son will not allow it.
Very religious. Worships and
fasts. Made pilgrimage.
Sees well, deaf in 1 ear,
speaks loudly.
Never been sick, never had
pills or drugs.
Eats milk, yogurt, fruit,
nuts, butter, bread,
skim milk, and occasionally
meat.
Smokes 6 cigarettes daily.
Drinks tea when tired.
Eats 3 times daily.
A farmer. Walks to town.
Hasn't worked in 23 years.
He is able, but his sons will
not allow it.
Happy and joyous.
Wants to live longer.

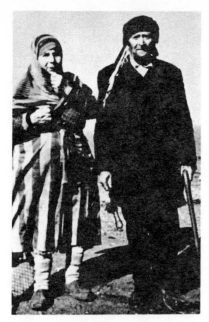

ABDULLAH SERIN:
103 years of age.
[With his wife.]

Sees poorly, a little deaf.
Eats all kinds of food.
Religious man. Worships
5 times daily.
Fasts in Ramadan.
When young, worked in the
fields.
Last year doctors told him not
to work too hard.
Married twice.
Has 3 sons, 1 daughter.

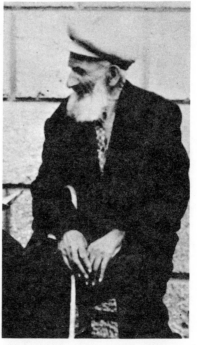

ZINE: 135 years of age.

Died in 1967.
Ate yogurt, milk and
vegetables.
Up to his death was always
active. Walked a lot.
Religious man with
conservative habits.

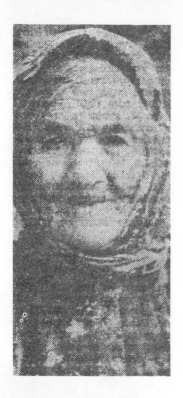

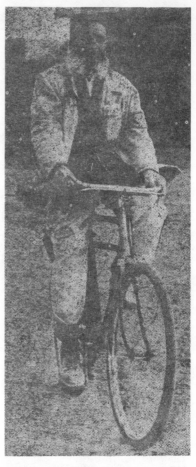

MAHMUT SAHIN NINE:
120 years of age.

District's oldest, but healthiest grandmother.
Afraid of towns and cities.
Has visited only 3 nearby villages.
Says people going to cities are all sick.
Claims she's never been sick.
Intends to stay well and reach 150 years of age.

SIRALI PARYAT ZEMCANT:
117 years of age.

Lives in Erdebil.
Married 17 times.
Youngest wife was 13 and oldest was 40.
Now has 4 wives living in different homes.
Hard-working, merry man.
Sells materials for buildings in village. Works like a young man.
Never smoked and does not drink. Says this is the reason for his robust, long and healthy life.

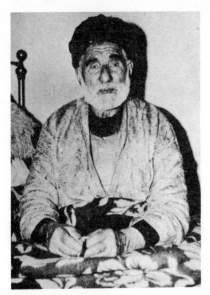

ALI ASKER HUSEYINI:
110 years of age.

Born in Iran.
Came to Turkey at 18.
Likes yogurt, milk, honey,
butter, all fruits.
Married only once
Hasn't smoked or drunk tea
in 60 years.
Usually drinks milk.
Very religious. Worships
5 times daily. Fasts 3 months
a year, during Ramadan and
2 months before.
After 40, began to read many
books about religion.
Knows Russian and Persian
languages.
Cannot hear or see well.
After eyes examined 2 years
ago, he used lemon on them
instead of doctor's
prescription.
Brave and courageous.
Not even afraid of dying.
Before 40 worked in fields
and was a shepherd also.
Walks for an hour every day.

IRAN

When we traveled, one of my
main objectives in seeking
some of these elderly people
was to meet the oldest and to
see what changes were taking
place.
We heard of a man who was
well over 150 years of age in
Iran and although we chased
all over the country to find
him, spending considerable
time and effort, we were not
fortunate enough to locate
him.
However, there were several
old men we did find in Iran,
but it was believed that they
were of Turkish descent.

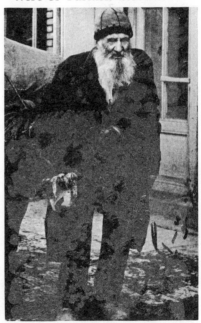

HACI ALI IKZEMASAZ:
120 years old.

Traveled for 26 years
in Syria and Arabia.
He is from Iran.

RAMADAN

Ramadan is the holy month of the Moslems. To commemorate this, able-bodied Moslems fast during Ramadan. From daybreak to sunset they do not eat or drink. After sundown they may partake of food in moderation. This is an important point because moderation is one of the World Keys.

SOMETHING TO THINK ABOUT

How old is old? Christian Jacobsen Dranberg, a Dane, was born in 1626 and died in 1772 at 146! At the age of 70 he was taken prisoner by Algerian pirates. He served as a slave for 15 years, then escaped and participated in a war against Sweden. At the age of 111, the Dane married a woman of 60 and outlived her. At 130 he proposed to several women but was rejected. He lived another 16 years, during which his conduct was "far from blameless", but he simmered down at the age of 141 and died at 146.

"If one man can live a life as full as this," said Dr. Theodore Klumpp of New York City, "there is no reason why science cannot make it possible for many of us to marry at 111, propose and be accepted at 130 and live to 146. Middle aged people should not prepare to be old, then they could take the aging process as it comes instead of hurrying toward it.

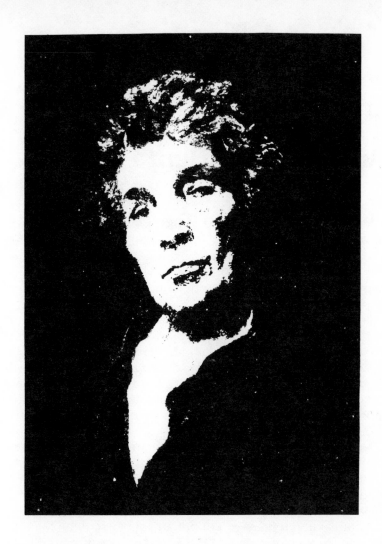

PETER MARTIN AT THE AGE OF 185 YEARS

One of the most remarkable examples of longevity of any man of modern times was a Hungarian. Simple in life and habits, an observance of natural diet, drink, sleep, good will to all mankind, and such exercise as keep the spine normal, would make the average life 100 years or more.

For long life, avoid vaccinations, serums, poison medicines, intoxicants, tobaccos, all stimulants and narcotics, high-heeled shoes or boots, tight belts and corsets, and revelings of all kinds. Live naturally and without anxiety, eat, drink, and sleep well, keep the body and mind clean, and serve God and humanity.

Chapter 7

Arriving in the Hunza Valley

Visiting the legendary land of the Hunzas fulfilled a dream of over 35 years. We had heard many stories about this area and now we had the chance to explore for ourselves. One of the highlights was staying in the palace with the King, Mohammed Jamal Khan, the Mir of Hunza, his family and meeting the gracious citizens of this Valley.

En route we stopped in Gilget, Pakistan's most important northern outpost where our party picked up jeeps and guides. We were warned by the guide that the roads and bridges have been washed out many times by rushing waters flowing from the glaciers and there was danger of sudden rock slides. As we traveled 64 miles over treacherous roads, which were little more than a ledge, we were well aware of the frequent drops of 2,000 feet.

Midway in our descent we met hardy mountain people, both men and women, who despite their ages are able to climb like goats over rocky inclines while carrying heavy loads. Gifts of fruit welcomed us as we entered the Hunza Valley. We were greeted by the men only as the women do not appear in public. Word of our arrival reached the Mir and he made us welcome. When he invited us to stay at his palace he expressed the thought that he would be only too glad to help us in any way possible. We stayed at the new palace, built 25 years ago by the present Mir's father. New, because the former one was built 600 years ago!

HISTORY OF THE PEOPLE

The Mir was very interested in diet and nutrition and during the 8 days we spent at the palace we talked extensively on diet and proper care of the body. He is interested in natural culture and in preserving it as much as possible among his people. He realized the difficulty of carrying on with life as in the past while the influence of city life is coming into their beautiful valley.

However, I do believe the health of the Hunzas, on the average, is much better than most countries of the world. They have every reason to be healthier because of their climate, their altitude and being forced to live in primitive ways. Until recent times, these people have been locked in the Hunza Valley for centuries where no outside influences could affect them. Nine months of the year they were closed in their valley due to weather conditions and could only travel when the passes were open the remaining three months.

The Mir told us there is no written history but over 2,000 years ago a few soldiers left the army of Alexander the Great to settle here with their Persian wives. When Alexander the Great went east from Macedonia he took with him the strong people of the Balkan States, Iran, Turkey and what is now Southern Russia. The strongest men of those countries comprised his army. In our travels we found the strongest and most elderly people still live in this section of the world. It is said that the Mir of Hunza is a descendent of Alexander the Great and we see the lion, Alexander's mark, in their flag.

The early descendents of the soldiers brought their inherent strength and culture from their homelands. Many in this valley have the blue eyes which is not usual for this region. The people still have some of the same habits and customs; all the dances are done by the men and are similar to the ancient Persian ones. The hard, bony, calcium structure of their bodies is very evident.

FAMOUS HUNZA APRICOTS

And, we include the famous Hunza apricots! The apricot originated in the central part of Europe and moved east to Greece and Turkey. It's in this area also that grapes grow well and grapes grow very well indeed in the Hunza Valley as it compares a good deal to the climate, altitude, and surroundings of Turkey and the lower part of Russia.

I noticed that most of the apricot trees were tall and spread out and I asked about the ages of them and was told that many of the trees were over one hundred years old. These famous Hunza apricots are deserving of their reputation for sweetness and flavor. The abundance of the fruit makes it a staple and the kernel of the apricot seed is a prime source of protein.

Now, proteins are the greatest of all foods to give stimulation to the heart and glands, but when you live in the higher altitudes you cannot have too many stimulating foods in your diet. The apricot, while high in protein, is like the almond and does not produce extreme stimulation to the heart structure. These people did a lot of climbing and were very nimble. They did not have heart troubles to speak of, nor were they short-winded.

The bitter kernels are made into oils and the sweet ones are directly eaten. A delicacy that is said to have great healing power is the apricot drink made by rubbing dried apricots in a bowl of water until the fruit is dissolved into a thick drink. This is the "Chamus" which is included in our recipe section.

SPRING PLANTING AND THE LAND

The coming of spring always brings new life to the Hunza Valley and planting starts as soon as possible with ceremonies for both the planting and sowing. The land has always been their life. It provides food, fuel and fabric for the people. Their ancestors cleared the stones from the fields and used them to build homes and canals for waterways.

ROCKS AND WATER

Piles of rocks are wherever you go. The homes are built of rock, as well as the flumes, and roadways. In the past they had no implements to work with and they just used the ibex horn as a pick ax. Our translator explained how they did this: For breaking big boulders, first of all they lit a big fire on top of it, then they poured cold water on it and then took big stones and smashed it into pieces. Now with modern means it is easy, but in the past they must have been giants, in their strength and courage.

Their irrigation channels are a work of art and engineering skill and their flumes cover an area of 17,000 sq. miles. There is very little rainfall, about 25 inches a year, but they get water from the glacier constantly. Water is their blood. It is everything they have. Without water it is not possible for any animal to exist. It would all be desert if it wasn't for the running water. Remember the Persian saying "If you can bring water to the desert you can get a rose to bloom" and they certainly had beautiful vegetation.

Even though their farming methods are primitive, they have preserved the delicate balance of soil, plant and animal life. The Hunza farmer practices crop rotation, and returns all human, animal and vegetable matter to the soil. No artificial fertilizer is allowed. While most of the ground in the Hunza

Valley is terraced, very hilly and hard to get to, you have to be in good condition to go from one section to another. They have their terraced gardens right to the edge of the cliffs that go directly into the Hunza River. No ground is wasted; they use every bit of soil possible. This is one reason why they do not have animals very much in the Valley. They cannot afford to keep animals as they eat far more food than humans do and the protein return doesn't pay.

One of the scientists summed up the simple way of these people. "They live in two-storied houses almost all the same size with walls of stone and mud with a flat roof. The first floor is for livestock, the second floor is for living space divided into a closed room and an open veranda. The veranda is used in summer as it is cool there. The other room is completely closed except for one small entrance and a chimney hole. Hence, no sunlight can enter. In winter all the family gather in this room which may be warmed by a fire, but there is nothing to prevent smoke damage or infection by disease."

DIET AND FOODS

Two meals a day are eaten and much of their food is taken raw. Their diet includes plenty of raw vegetables such as turnips, carrots, peas, spinach, green leafy vegetables and fruits; dried apricots, apples, pears, cherries and mulberries.

Both fruits and vegetables are sun dried for later use. They have an adequate amount of carbohydrates in their millet, buckwheat, barley, rye and corn. Their protein intake is low, as compared to the protein intake of the elderly people we found in the Caucasus and Azerbaijan areas, however they do have beans, peas and nuts; almonds, walnuts, and the apricot kernel. There is very little milk due to the lack of pasturage for animals. Their dairy products are derived chiefly from sheep and goats plus milk and yogurt are used. There is very little poultry or eggs as the chickens eat the seeds for their crops. They have meat only during the winter months and in small quantities. There are wild sheep, some beef and mutton, but all in limited supply. Fats and oils are short in measure; however, they do use the apricot oil for culinary purposes and some milk is converted into butter. Linseed oil is used also.

The question of fats has been a big one in the past. It was believed that the calories counted more than the components of the diet and the absence or presence of fats hardly mattered. The classical work of Burr and Burr in 1929, however, revolutionized this concept and brought home the fact that certain unsaturated fatty acids are not only essential for growth but for survival also.

Cereals provide the bulk and calories in the Hunza diet— about 52%. Weight for weight, consumption of fruit is greater than that of cereals. They serve many unusual dishes in their natural form which I am sure has been conducive to building good bodies and good health. When in season, the fruit is sun-dried and converted into flour or used in their natural dried fruit form. Many times they put apricot kernels in the dried fruit, using it as a soup which is considered a delicacy. A delicious treat are their dried mulberries which are also ground and made into flour.

THRESHING GRAIN

The Hunza method of threshing is by using donkeys to tread on the grain and separate it from the chaff. The donkey then carries the grain to the little one room mills where the farmers may grind their grain, free of charge. Only whole grain is used in Hunza bread and is made available by means of stone grinding, which does not heat the seeds and therefore the flour isn't damaged.

RECIPES

Some interesting recipes for beverages of the Hunza:

KHANDA

Mulberry fruit juice prepared by cooking dried mulberries in an excess of water for 30 to 60 minutes.

SATOO

3 lb. Dried Apple Flour
1 lb. Sprouted Wheat Flour
Water is added to the mixture and it is served cold as a refreshing drink.

DAODO

1 lb. Apricot Flour
1 lb. Sprouted Wheat Flour
Mixture is added to water and served as a cold drink.

CHAMUS

Dried apricots are washed in water until they have been completely dissolved.

They have a food called Saapinder, which is served only on very special occasions. This is made from butter oil and stored in stoneware for as long as forty years. They claim it has great healing power. I understand it is quite offensive to the taste, but it is considered a great delicacy.

Other local food recipes:

DIRAMSPIK

1 lb. Sprouted Wheat Flour
4 lb. Unsprouted Wheat Flour

CHAPATIS

Made from the above mixture and fried in butter oil, walnut oil, apricot oil or deep fat.

BERRYKUZ

Stuffed Chapatis are prepared by mixing dough with spiced apricot nut flour and are fried in the seed oil.

HAWALOO-GARAMAMUCH

1 lb. Bread Crumbs
3 lbs. Spinach Leaves
½ lbs. Apricot Nut Powder
½ lb. Onions

The spinach leaves are cooked with the onions, red chili and apricot nut powder. Bread crumbs are added to cooked spinach leaves and food is eaten as such.

MALEEDA

Bread Crumbs are fried in butter oil or apricot oil and mixed with whey, salt and spices. Mixture is cooked until it becomes thick.

It was a wonderful sight to see these people living in the natural beauty of nature, and living in the purities found in the primitive state. It would have been more or less easy to have balanced their diets by adding some greens—more of the chlorophyl foods. Most of the problems which were brought to my attention could be cared for by the addition of the green foods, which would give them the extra Vitamin A so necessary to a diet.

Malva is one of the most plentiful plants growing in Hunza Valley. It is one of the greens having a great amount of Vitamin A and would be of great value to them.

FOODS

One of the most abundant of all the foods served was their home-pounded cereal grains, which they had made into Chapatis. This gives them a good amount of Vitamin B, also.

When their food was analyzed it was found that there is sufficient amounts of potassium, calcium, and sodium in their diet. The iron content may be somewhat less than in many others, but living at this high altitude, the blood count is always high.

HEALTH OF THE HUNZAS IS TESTED

Scientists who have visited claim that this is not a Utopia free of any disease whatsoever, however they do believe that many of the diseases they have today appeared within the last 50 years. They claim that the hard labor the Hunzas are forced to undertake and the lack of mental stress is bound to influence their health. Statistics showed that in the last thousand years only 10 % of the people ever left the valley, and none of the people above the age of 60 who were examined had hypertension. Arteriosclerosis seems almost absent from the tests.

HEALTH OF HUNZAS

They have a blood pressure that ranges from 110 to 155 with a diastolic from 70 to 110. Electrocardiograms prove that they have been found to be healthier than average. The doctors advise that an increase in milk products would insure better protein nutrition, especially of the children. It was only those who had the extra money and could afford a little extra meat who had the sufficient amount of protein that these scientists thought was necessary. They did note that not a single member of the population was overweight. The Hunza people they found, did have the proper amount of calcium in their diets. And it is well to know that their mulberries and the mulberry flour were very high in calcium and potassium while the fenugreek bread was very high in sodium, potassium and calcium. As a rule, they have a good blood count and good calcium metabolism due to the altitude and climate. Their mineral water intake is good and they get enough ultra violet. In general, the Hunzas seem to possess remarkably good health.

The fast moving glacial water carries a fine silt, rich in minerals. Although it is unappealing in appearance, this muddy glacial water is drunk in abundance by the Hunzakuts. I am sure that many of the minerals these people get for use in their bodies are found in these glacial waters, and I am sure that these waters make the land and soil fertile. The Mir preferred to personally use the muddy glacial waters—heavy with silt, while he insisted on serving us a pure spring water.

Goiter has been quite prevalent in this country, but is disappearing. In some villages there were many cases of this disease, and in others, none. A reason for this could be that they had struck a crater in the glacial water that could be bringing iodine into the valley.

When we inquired about the health problems of the people the Mir told us that there were many suffering from eye troubles especially in the summertime, though not many were bothered by this problem in the winter. They do have a lot of windstorms and from the lack of rain the turned over soil seems to blow into a fine dust. This fine dust storm may stay for days and seems to encourage eye troubles.

I told the Mir of Hunza how the malva growing wild was a nourishing food, high in Vitamin A, and he surprised us one night at dinner and served cooked malva. It was very good, nice and green, his cook did a wonderful job. It wasn't seasoned and tasted like spinach.

We also mentioned to them about making tea and showed you can take the alfalfa and peppermint growing in the fields and make tea instead of using the black teas. They do have green tea from China, but they put sugar in this and spices and we explained how honey is better.

INTERPRETER

I asked our interpreter if the advent of civilization wasn't cutting down on the good health and the life of these people and he said "Yes, this is true. By coming into contact with civilization one gains something and one loses something." According to him, they were probably losing more than they were gaining. "For instance, we have lost many things and one of them is our health foods that are grown in our valley." He told me that in the past there was no market for their fresh fruits and all that was produced was consumed by the people there. There was now a ready market for their foods in Rawalpindi and in Gilgit and other cities, so now instead of consuming their beautiful fresh foods they take them to the cities to sell and trade for tea, coffee, white sugar and cigarettes and are spoiling their health. By coming into contact with civilization a man may acquire manifold so-called "necessities", but often his income may not increase proportionately, and the most valuable thing he loses is his peace of mind.

He was telling us that in these civilized times people were

changing their attitudes. He mentioned that is was a custom, not in the far past, but in the time of his own remembrance that if you passed by an orchard, anyone who was there would take you by the arm, invite you in and offer you the available food. If you refused, he was offended. "Now comes a time when even your friend will turn his head away so he will not see you and have to offer you food. And all the trees you see growing on the other side of the road were free for anybody to help himself. The only thing was that you could go there and eat any quantity but you were not allowed to take it home, because in that case a few could take the whole crop home. Today, they guard these trees, so that man in his greed would not pick them."

When people lived simply their necessities were very few. Food for the whole year, clothes to cover the body and protection from heat and cold and a small house; these were the only things one required. In the past unusual stories of their radiant health and long life have been recorded and while they still live close to nature many of their natural foods are being traded off for a "mess of pottage". The King is well aware of this but is unable to stop it. Much of their cultural background is breaking up since the advent of the jeep, warfare and the population explosion. The men must join the army and they bring back the diseases of civilization and the changes from the outside world.

They want automobiles, they want to drive a jeep, they want to have some of the comforts of the wealthy—these are the goals and ideals of life. It is the old men who tell you that the food routine has changed. It is the elderly who see what has happened to their natural past and who lament the new habits that are beginning to come into their valley.

OLD PEOPLE

Of course we came to see the heroes of Hunza—the old men! Longevity has been a reality here to the degree that there are a great number of healthy people between the ages of 70 and 100. One of the elderly patriarchs of 110 years of age, left his work in the fields and walked 2 miles to meet me. He still walked with amazing briskness.

I visited several groups of elders and was very impressed with their bodily strength and endurance. They lived by our Keys of Exercise and Activity as well as many of the others. I found them limber and vital. Whenever possible I shook hands with the old men in order to feel the strength of their handclasp. Strength and flexibility was truly theirs. I met a man of 72 and was told he was very active in a responsible job as a chief engineer of roads in Hunza. His hands were like those of a young man.

Just outside the village of Schalt, I met the oldest man I could find in Hunza. He was 120, and a devout believer in the simple natural way of living. As was my practice in other countries, I collected a few strands of his beard for analysis.

I asked how the age of the old men could be determined and although one man did not know the date of his birth he could relate it in this way, "In 1892 when we were conquered by the British I was a boy and played polo on foot." We can then surmise that he is over 90 years of age.

There were very few over 120 now because of the habits they are adopting. As one of the old men said, "Once it was usual for everyone to awaken when the sky was full of stars, in the morning, to say our prayers. By the time we had finished our prayers there would still be stars in the sky. We went to bed very early and took very simple foods; fruits, vegetables and we are simple in our habits and eat plenty. We do not think it unusual to be in good health or to live to a very old age."

POLO

Polo is a favorite sport, but when played Hunza style is close to warfare! The Hunzakuts are considered to be among the world's finest polo players. Every village had a polo ground where everyone participated. It was a very rough game in the past and your life was at stake! It was not unusual for 4 or 5 persons in the village to die at each game and wounds were very common. It was a manly game!

Since the coming of the jeeps and vehicles it is not economical for a poor person to keep a horse so that they are disappearing. They are constructing schools and mosques in the center of those fields and we observed that there was not one standard size for these polo grounds because of the shortage of flat land. They made use of whatever land was available.

Previously, there was only one kingdom but it was divided into Hunza and Nagir three or four centuries ago. There were two brothers who couldn't get along and they were each given one side of the valley to rule. In spite of the fact that people on both sides are related there was constant quarreling until 1892 when the British came in and peace has prevailed since then.

When we visited with the Mir of Nagir and his family my wife, Marie, had a long lovely visit with the Princess, the Mir of Nagir's daughter who was about to be married. I welcomed this opportunity to hear more about their customs, for since my arrival I was avoided by the women; they all turned their eyes down when I entered a room. When I asked my interpreter about the veils the women wore and about their shyness, he said that it was a religious rule that while you moved about you did not gaze into women's faces, you kept your eyes down. The same order applies to the women. "It is not that our religion orders us to keep our women inside and put them away, but to keep your eyes down." The veil, I believe comes from the Hindus.

Marie: "Of course, I had a lot of questions and so did the Princess. The Princess was interested in nutrition and what foods were good to eat. I told her it was best to leave out the white sugar with their teas (as they use a great deal of this) and I explained to them about using raw shredded salads with dressing and went into more detail about recipes.

The Queen was so grateful for my information that she gave me two embroidered bands to go around the cuffs of sweaters and in the front. They are beautifully done and it takes a long time, but they have many cold winter nights to do this.

The Princess was going to be married in a red wedding dress because this is a sign of happiness. It was a beautiful gown and it had about a 6″ band of needlework, to wear around her forehead and tie in the back with two long streamers down each side with tassels—of all different colors. These are embedded in a gold filigree holder. I happened to have a little pin along and I gave it to the bride-to-be and told her if I had known she was getting married I would have brought her a nice gift. She was very happy. Of course, our jewelry is very different from theirs and this pleased her."

The Hunza women make their own clothes also and use lovely clear colors in their garments. Men weave as well as the women. The citizens usually have one set of clothes in winter, and their choga coat serves as overcoat and blanket. Customarily, women do not mix with men in public. This even holds true for the little girls who have their own separate school house. The boys attend school until the equivalent of our 12th grade but the girls do not have to go unless they wish. Although they may never contact the outside world, they have the opportunity to learn other languages and are taught Urdu and English.

FASTING

Fasting is also observed during the Moslem holy month of Ramadan. Food is only eaten between 8 o'clock at night and 2 o'clock in the morning. There is no smoking, drinking (even of water) and as our interpreter explained, they are ordered to see that "all our limbs are fasting, meaning you don't go any-place to do something bad or commit a sin. Your eyes must be fasting, you don't see something bad. Your mouth must be fasting, you don't say something wicked. And so every limb of your body must be fasting, otherwise it is quite useless."

Most of the population are Moslems and homage is paid by bowing in prayer five times a day. Every detail of their family life is under the control of religion. They are forbidden any kind of wine, or intoxicating drink.

BROTHERHOOD AND JUSTICE

A feeling of genuine brotherhood still prevails in this coun-try. There are no crimes, so there are no police or jails. How-ever, when disputes do arise, they are settled at daily council meetings. The Mir presides over the sessions which are com-prised of elders representing various villages.

Each case is discussed and put to vote, but the Mir has the final say. "Justice delayed, is justice denied." Here you saw a case decided within 5 minutes. The party who won the case would be elated and the other party, if they did not think the decision was fair can gather witnesses and consult their learned people about it. If these counsellors think the deci-sion was unfair the case can appear again before the court. If it is again decided against them, it is finished.

The Mir told us that there is always enough for everyone to eat and clothing to wear and there never seems to be a short-age. They all share.

Finally, it was time to say goodbye to our friends the Mir and his family. Staying with the Mir in his palace was one of our greatest experiences. He is very affable and truly a gentle-man that everyone in the Hunza Valley respects. The Mir was thrilled and extremely pleased with the honorary life mem-bership plaque I presented to him on behalf of the National Health Federation.

As I prepared to leave Hunza I reflected on the many years I searched for *that* valley of eternal youth, and now I realize that the Shangri La is in our consciousness. But in Hunzaland, I found a philosophy for living a long life which the Mir expressed so well. He told us that his belief is in Eternal Happiness and Peace; good international feelings; living close to nature and living on pure foods.

Welcome to Hunzaland [in Color]

Shangri-La, The Land of Terraces, Good Health and Long Life.

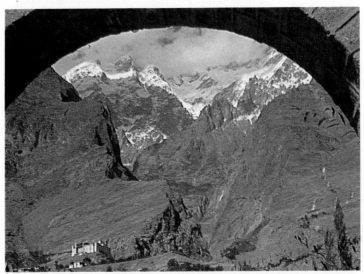

600-year-old castle that ruled Hunza before modern palace was built.

The King and I.

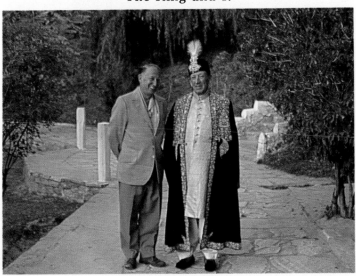

Color Section A

Welcome to Hunzaland

Hunzakut commune beneath Mt. Rakaposhi, 25,550 feet above sea level.

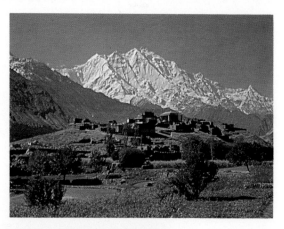

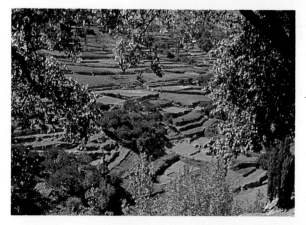

Hunzaland, the country of terraces.

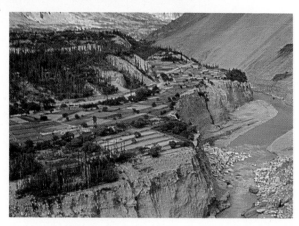

Color Section B

Welcome to Hunzaland

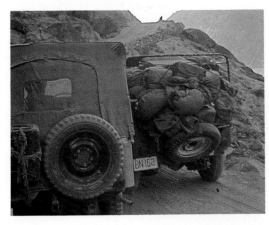

We were packed for the rough trip ahead.

Mountain men.

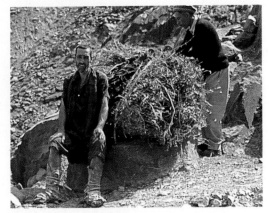

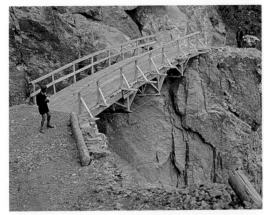

Bridge just finished for our travel through on the dangerous road to Hunza.

Welcome to Hunzaland

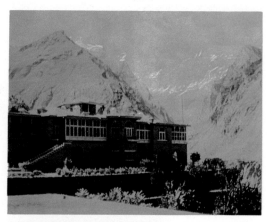

Hunza beauty in the moonlight and the Mirs Palace.

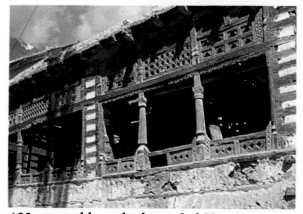

600-year-old castle that ruled Hunza before modern palace was built.

Classroom scenes.

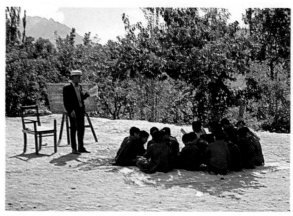

Color Section D

Welcome to Hunzaland

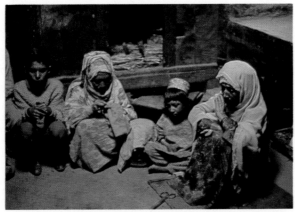

A family scene in their living room.

Children come by a good inheritance in Hunza.

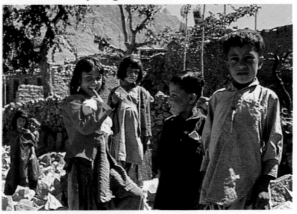

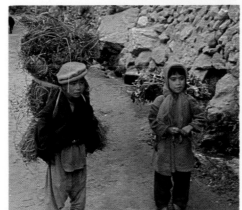

Everyone works in Hunza, even the children.

Color Section E

Welcome to Hunzaland

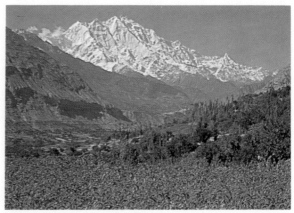

Millet fields in Hunza, a grain high in protein.

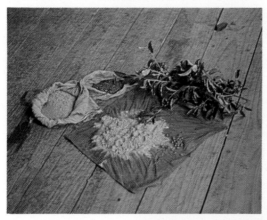

Buckwheat from the berry and the grain.

Separating the chaff from the grain with walking burros.

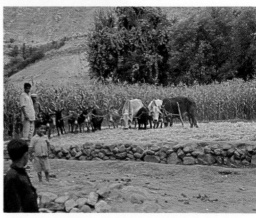

Welcome to Hunzaland

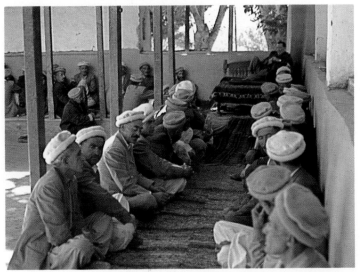

They hold court every morning at 10 o'clock.

110-year-old Hunzakut.

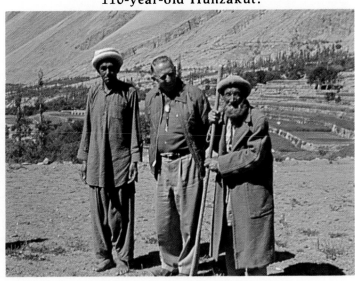

Color Section G

Welcome to Hunzaland

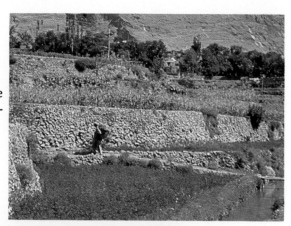

Hunzaland, the country of terraces.

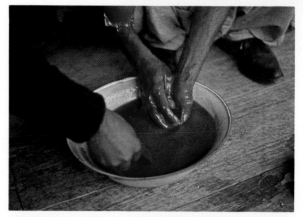

Making a juice from the dried apricots, rubbed and dissolved in water.

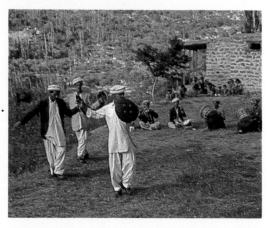

Dance and music.

Color Section H

Welcome to Hunzaland

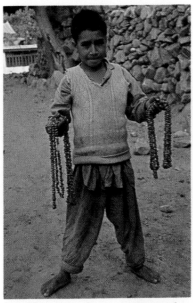

In Hunza they string the apricot kernels and eat them when hungry.

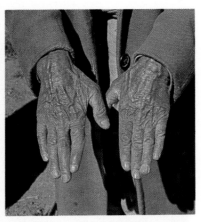

110-year-old hands, no arthritis or stiffness.

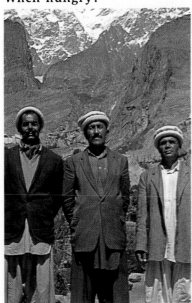

Hardy men to match their mountains.

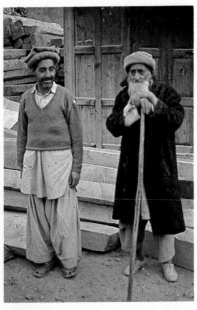

120-year-old Hunzakut with 65-year-old son.

The Elderly People

I have met all except Li Ching Yun and Thomas Parr.

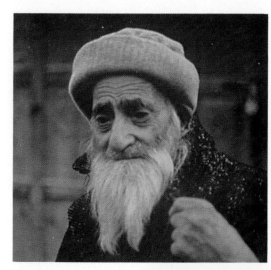

Hunzakut, 120 years old from Hunzaland, West Pakistan. He was in best of health when I last saw him.

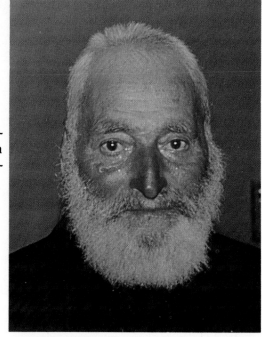

Mr. Gasanov, 153-year-old man from Russia whom I visited.

Color Section J

The Elderly People

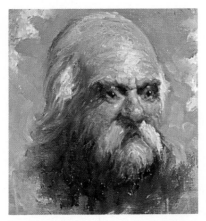

Li Ching Yun from Szechuan, China, 256 years of age— died 1930.

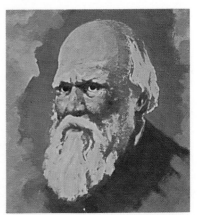

Thomas Parr, 153 years of age.

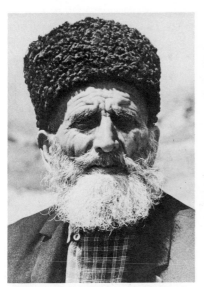

Shirali Muslimov of Russia, 167 years old.

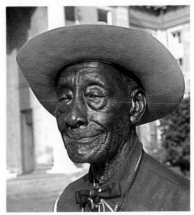

Charlie Smith, 133 years of age in Florida.

Color Section K

The Elderly People

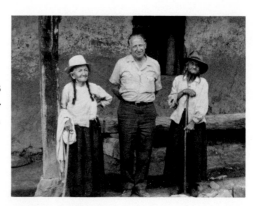

Two ladies, 100 years of age each, in Vilcabamba, Equador So. America.

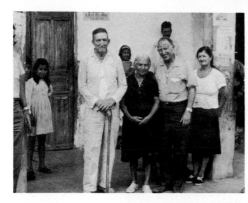

Carpio of Vilcabamba, 132 years old. Another man visited in this village was 140 years old.

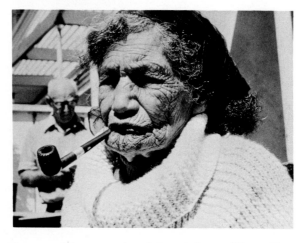

Granny Nga, native Maori from New Zealand.

Color Section L

INTRODUCTION TO KEYS

In the following section on the "World Keys to Health and Long Life" we are including photographs as illustrations along with the text.

We are starting out with two Keys: Beauty in Color, Music and Art, and Harmony and Balance. Although these Keys are presented better with the addition of color, they are not necessarily considered the most important.

The Keys are numbered according to their importance as I see it, both for good health and for the prolongation of life.

Color Section M

Beauty in Color, Music and Art

KEY # 18

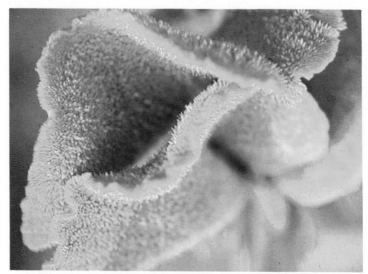

Beauty feeds the aesthetic nature of a person.

The feathers of a parrot. Beauty is distributed throughout all of nature.

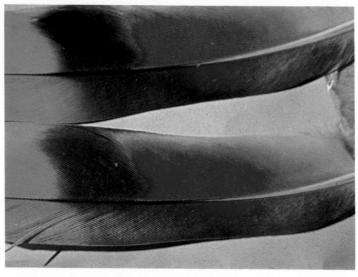

Beauty in Color, Music and Art

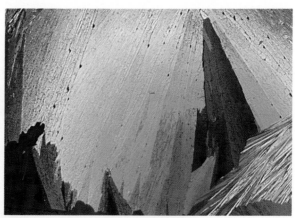

Crystals under a microscope. All of nature is composed of beautiful colors in its finite form.

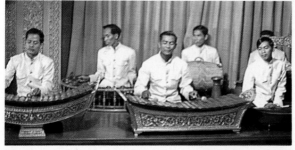

Thai orchestra communicating an uplifting note through music.

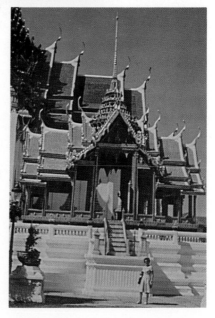

Temples of Thailand. Beauty as a creation is found in architecture.

Harmony and Balance

KEY #19

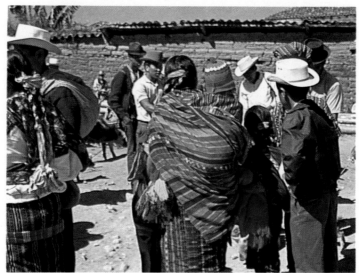

The people of Guatamala live balanced daily lives.

Nature brings balance through its expression of electrical storms and thunder to purify the air and brings the hue to the sunset.

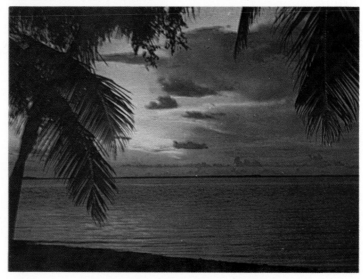

Color Section P

World Keys to Health and Long Life

Speaking about the World Keys, we are going to go through each key separately and discuss them briefly. However, we will go into them further throughout the text.

In going through all the different countries to find the keys that keep a person well, healthy, joyous, happy and living a long life, I find this one thing is true: that those who live the longest life are those who develop the greatest amount of activity, physically, mentally and spiritually. When I said activity, I mean that they develop every department of life. They go into parts of life that many other people never even think of, never even work with. I find as they begin to develop all the different departments of life, there is no need for treatments. There is no need for remedies, because they are living them. They are constantly using remedies that make their bodies well. They are constantly living a life that is treating them to the very best so that they can have a long life and good health.

Accomplishments are not everything in life, but whatever these people accomplish in life is done according to nature and is close to nature. So, they are accomplishing a great deal for themselves. Many people in civilization today are accomplishing things for other people. Many times we would lay down our life for another person. There is no need to do this. While these people do things for themselves, everybody else is doing it also. We don't find that individuals are expected to carry the whole burden, as we do in civilized life and in the city. There are many people who carry more of a burden than other people. Some are educated to carry a bigger burden.

These people who live a long life have no schooling. They haven't anything to unlearn. The only thing they really know is what nature produces for them, and they

117

live very close to nature. Nature preserves them in good health, as we all know, through good food, pure air, sunshine and unpolluted waters. All this purity is found with these people who live a long life and a happy one. When we see these long-lived people, they are as happy as they could be in their accomplishments. There is a possibility that people accomplish things in the city, and some who live a short life probably have touched a bit of happiness that those who have lived a long life will never touch. I feel it is not a matter of how long you live. I don't think a long life lived is good enough, but a good life lived is long enough.

One of these days we will view a man's life by what he has accomplished. After all, if there is only one life, an eternal one, it's a matter of growth. We go on from where we leave off. Our accomplishment is going to be what we have left behind as a heritage for others to live by, whether humanity is better for our coming this way, whether humanity needed us when we came this way, and whether God gives His approval on how we lived.

In this country, less than 3% of the doctors practice preventive medicine; yet this is what keeps people well. This is not a system of waiting for you to get sick and then doing something for you. Preventive medicine is making sure that the horse is taken care of before the barn door is left open—before you get the disease, and when the resistance is gone in your body and you are subject to a cold or flu. You're not even going to get into this position with a little prevention.

The people who live the longest life live in a state of complete prevention of disease. They don't walk into troubles. They live a life where they don't have to worry about disease. Those who have no disease and live the longest life have no doctors. They have beautiful teeth, and still have all their teeth when they die at 120 years of age. They are living in a preventive atmosphere; they are living a preventive life. This, in itself, is a great ideal and example for us to strive for.

We mention these KEYS only to awaken us. They are only here to make us think and have us realize that there is something beyond just taking some food or having a good time. There are definite laws that mankind has to follow. There are feelings the mind has to get acquainted with. There is a path man must travel. There are things he should know. I believe if a man knew just three principles he could keep out of most of his troubles.

First, he needs *knowledge.* Then he needs *wisdom,* and then he needs *guidance.* With these three things he can keep well, prevent disease, live a long life, get along with people, and fulfill these few world keys that follow.

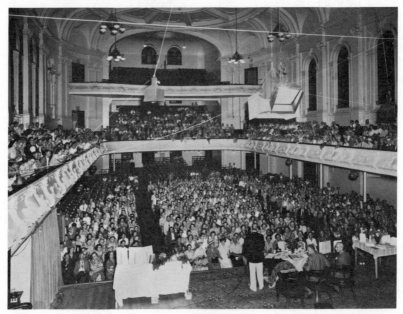

In some of our travels around the world we taught classes in other countries. Here, in Auckland, New Zealand we are teaching a class of 2,700 people how to live a happy, healthy, long life.

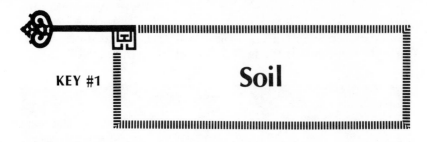

Soil

Soil has been misunderstood for a long time. We should recognize that the soil is the giver of life. I spent time in a little monastery in the southern part of Russia where one of the monks was telling me that the earth was originally called Mother Earth because she gave everything she could to her children, and her children's happiness was dependent upon the food she provided. She provided her children with water and minerals, with fruits, vegetables and shade from the trees. She gave everything that was needed, and this is why she was called Mother Earth.

Today we don't realize the value of Mother Earth. We have plundered the earth. We have prostituted the earth. We have taken from the earth and we haven't followed the idea the Good Book gives us that we must replenish the earth. We are takers. We haven't been giving back to the earth and to the soil the replenishment that is necessary so our natural resources can be taken care of properly.

It has been said, that 85 years ago there was some 80 inches of topsoil throughout the United States. Today the government tells us there is less than 8 inches on the average throughout the United States. We grow our vegetables from topsoil. Life comes from the topsoil.

Worm life lives in this topsoil. But the worms will not live in earth where artificial fertilizers or sprays have been used. Worms are migrators and will leave. Worms are necessary for aerating the soil. Very few know we cannot do without these lovely little monsters who take care of our life through keeping the soil active and giving it the bacterial possibilities where good food can grow.

One of the outstanding Keys is that we found no old men living where the soil was brown, dust-blown, or where there were no trees. We find all old men live where the soil is black. This is one thing the Mir of Hunza said

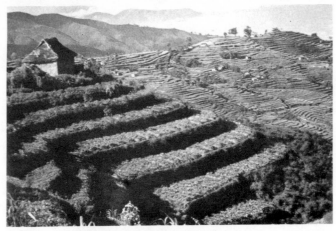

Terraces in Central America.

The Chinese save all their soil by building flat terraces which do not allow rivers and rain to carry it away.

The Hunzas save all of their soil as they need it to grow food for the family. It is the most precious thing they have. The Mir of Hunza told me that the oldest man lives where the soil was the blackest.

after I called it to his attention: "You know, all the old men live where the soil is blackest." I did not find old men in the South Seas where the water has carried away the topsoil. You do not see the topsoil in India because of a lack of water; and there is a lack of growth and a lack of the cycle of life taking place where growth would go back into the soil, bringing in humus and aerating it again; the

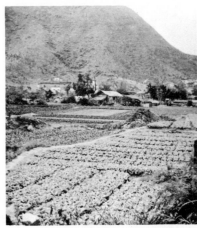

Aberdeen, China.
A farm scene.

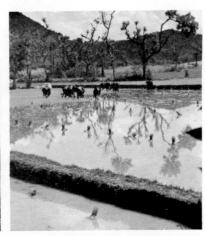

Bangkok, Thailand.
A rice paddy.

life cycle isn't there. Black soil is made through composting, where the dead material has returned to the earth. You find this is necessary. This is to awaken people to the fact that Mother Earth and the soil are very important to our life.

In the Caucasus valley in Russia, the soil is black as can be. In Turkey, where people live the long life, the soil is the blackest. Down in Vilcabamba, in South America, where they grow beautiful vegetables and fruits for their families, again the soil is black. It is in a valley made of topsoil—the dust of the earth from which man is made and which he needs so much.

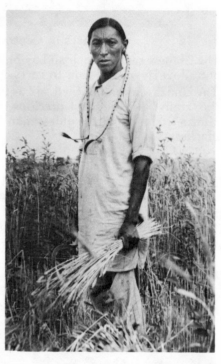

MAN NEEDS GOOD EARTH

It has been recorded that at one time "man was as tall as the cedars and as strong as the oaks". It was a time when man lived close to the earth, and a time when that earth was vital and young. It is said that "two men came out of the valley of Kadesh-Barnea carrying one bunch of grapes on a pole between them"! A wonderful bunch of grapes that were rich in life-giving, health-giving qualities imparted to them by a soil that was fertile and "alive". The kind of grapes that could build "men tall as cedars and strong as oaks"!

There are only a few places on the earth today where man lives a simple, natural life and maintains a healthy, hardy body. The Hunzas of West Pakistan are one of the few peoples left of the "Tall as Cedars and Strong as Oaks" races of men.

Today, particularly in the so-called "civilized" areas of the world, people are living off soil that is demineralized, devitalized, and so badly depleted that man is now a creature beset by physical ills and bedeviled by mental maladjustments. Man has consistently taken from the earth and not given in return. He has broken the spiritual law which demands he give in order to receive. Man, who should walk the earth like a king and be custodian of all he surveys, has degraded himself to the point where he is merely the despoiler of Nature. Nature, following the inexorable laws of life, takes her toll of man. Doctors find the vast majority of people are sadly lacking in minerals, mineral elements and vitamins. In short, they are suffering from MALNUTRITION.

Speaking of malnutrition, Dr. D. W. Cavanaugh of Cornell University stated, "There is only one major disease, and that is MALNUTRITION. All ailments and afflictions to which we may fall heir are directly traceable to this major disease."

It is time we realized that malnutrition goes deeper than just a bad combination of foods put together in our kitchens. It goes further than how you may cook the different elements out of your food by boiling, frying, and oversteaming. It goes further than eating food which has been standing around from four or five days to two weeks with a resultant loss of its chemical elements. It even goes further than what foods taste good and look good. In the natural course of events, tissues are broken down in the body and must be renewed. When you work you become tired and hungry; the body then reaches out for the element-building-blocks to appease your hunger and replace worn out tissues. If these element-building-blocks are not supplied through food, the body begins to slowly die from lack of replenishment. We recognize this as malnourishment or disease.

In a dying body you will have such ill-health symptoms as lack of appetite, abnormal cravings, pains, short breath, nervousness and a body that bruises easily.

It has been realized and recognized by many farmers, professors and doctors that the basic problem of getting an adequate mineral supply to our bodies through the natural fruit and vegetable kingdom can only be solved by a standard mineralized soil covering the range of minerals required by the body. This balanced soil would produce balanced bodies, or bodies free from malnutrition and disease. We know that 70 or more minerals are needed to maintain our bodies properly.

KNOWN ESSENTIAL ELEMENTS FOR THE ADEQUATE NUTRITION OF MAN

AIR ELEMENTS	TWELVE MAJOR MINERAL ELEMENTS	
Carbon	Chlorine	Phosphorus
Oxygen	Fluorine	Potassium
Hydrogen	Sodium	Magnesium
Nitrogen	Silicon	Manganese
	Calcium	Sulphur
	Iron	Iodine

TRACE MINERAL ELEMENTS

Cobalt	Cadmium	Barium
Aluminum	Mercury	Strontium
Zinc	Germanium	Titanium
Tin	Lead	Copper
Arsenic	Bromine	Zirconium
Vanadium	Boron	Cerium
Selenium	Nickel	Thorium
Beryllium	Lithium	Antimony
Silver	Ribidium	Bismuth
Gold	Caesium	Chromium

The genetic pattern itself has evolved certain chemical elements in the human body and in animals. The supply of these elements must be kept in the body through the soil. We obtain the minerals we need from plant life which subsists primarily upon the minerals obtained from the soil, plus the chemical action of the sun and nitrogen and carbon dioxide from the air. It takes certain minerals to grow more wool on an animal, and healthy hair on the human head; specific minerals are needed for the different organs of the body, the muscles and bones.

When we know that our circulation must have certain mineral elements to function, that the contractability of the arteries is maintained by certain elements, that the softness of the tissues and the strength and pliability of the muscle structure requires certain elements to keep in prime condition, then we know that we must look to the soil for help. When we consider that obesity, high-blood pressure, goiter and many other diseases can be avoided and overcome wholly by taking care of the desired mineral balance in the body, then it becomes a necessity that we start with the soil as the basis upon which we must build the foundation for good health.

Disease preys on the undernourished in nature just as it does in the human body. The General Manager of the Hidden Valley Health Ranch can look at an avocado tree and tell what elements are missing in the soil in which it is growing. When he sees the old leaves get brown and begin to turn up at the edges, he knows there is not enough boron in the soil.

At the University of Southern California's experimental station, all varieties of oranges go through their laboratories. They get perfect oranges and they get shrivelled up oranges with peelings that look as if they were suffering from psoriasis, the skin disease. These scientists, like my manager, can tell what kind of soil the different types of oranges came from and what is missing. The same holds true when I look at you. I can tell what is missing in your diet. That is the way I know when you have a disease.

ORGANIC GARDENING

There are people all over the country today planting organic gardens. Good food only comes from soil that has been properly cared for and composted to keep the mineral balance high. Celery, for instance, is much higher in minerals when grown on such soil than the regular grocery store variety. We must have this kind of food, because when we are lacking minerals and vitamins, we are on our way to dis-ease, ill health, ailments—all sorts of physical problems. Where did you think these came from? You are made from the dust of the earth. You gather up this dust of the earth with the vegetable and the fruit, and you mold it, as a sculptor does his clay, and build it into this human body. Indeed, we are wonderfully and fearfully made. We are not like an automobile made of steel and tin, needing only a bit of mineral out of the earth put through a heating process to turn out more steel for a new fender. We must replenish the materials the body is made of, but it is the life force working through the tissues that does the building and repair. Just as the root of the parsley plant goes down into the ground to draw out the minerals to make itself, so we have a root system in our bodies to take all that we need from food to build good skin structure, ears, hair and bowels, if the proper material is in that food. It is for this reason that we need greens, we need yellow vegetables, red fruits—all the colors Nature has given us. We need conscientious men tending our crops to make sure that the vegetable structure has the material in it. Along with this we have to have the wife, mother or cook to take care of the food in the kitchen, because in the kitchen the life-giving material can be so mutilated as to be useless for building health. Twenty-five per cent of the iron in foods is lost in cooking. We can't afford this loss because most of us are at least 25 % short of iron.

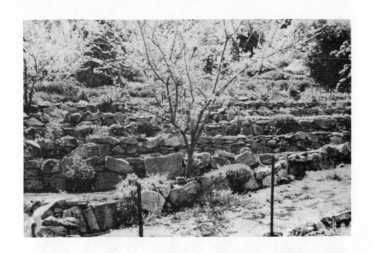

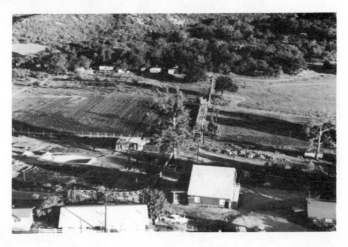

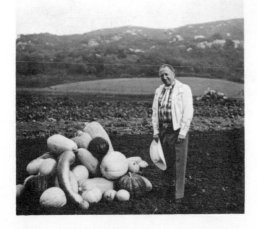

I have found on my Hidden Valley Health Ranch that black soil grows the best foods. When all that has been grown is returned to the soil, the natural composting helps to rebuild, aerate and keep it black.

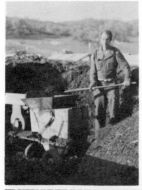

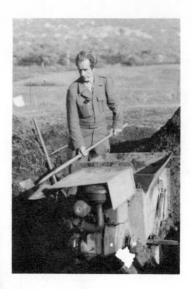

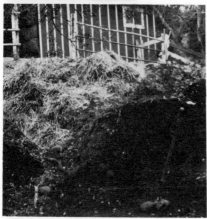

Making compost to replenish the earth.

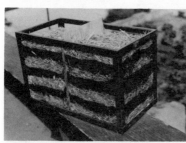

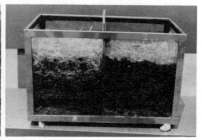

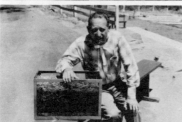

Experiment at Hidden Valley Health Ranch. This is how added worms break up soil. They are really man's best friend. This was done with soil and straw in two week's time.

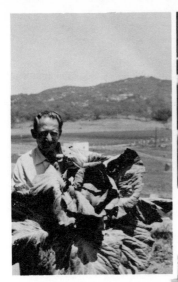

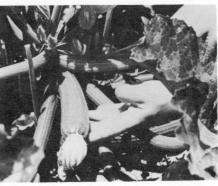

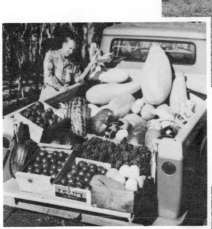

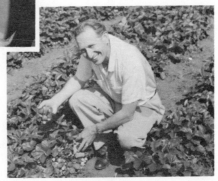

The soil is quite productive
when taken care of properly.

Temperance — The Greatest Key of All

I consider temperance the most important Key of all. I personally believe, after reading about the old men and visiting them and checking on their habits that they live a frugal life and one of economy. They practice a temperate life more than anything else.

Some of the old men were drinkers and drank whiskey every day. Some smoked all the time. The first elderly man I met in Turkey was 110 years of age and he came to see me with a cigarette in his mouth. I wanted to know how long he had been smoking, "Well, I started smoking at 90 years of age." I asked him why he started and he told me his children taught him. I wonder if this is going to cut down on his life.

There are elderly people who are heavy meat eaters and some who are light meat eaters and others who eat no meat at all and are vegetarians. I wondered what it really was that kept these people living the long life, and I believe it is because they are temperate. I would describe this as a state of "habitual moderation". They do not overdo, they do not go to extremes, they do not indulge in any excessive appetites.

I believe one of the greatest factors of all the Keys is that the elderly people ate very little, had small meals and many of them had only one meal a day. Many of them would drink at one time of the day and have their meal at another time. When they did eat, the portions were small.

One of the most important things we encountered was that they all followed the same pattern: the older they got, the less they ate.

There is an economy in our body, and I feel the moment we overeat or overindulge, we put the bodily energies to work in doing things they should not have to do. It is vital energy, whether it be brain force, brain energy, or muscular energy, that we find in time will wear out the body.

It is in their moderation, in their temperance and in their practice of staying away from many things that would tear down their bodies, that these old people are able to live this long life.

I might say that those who lived the longest lives were those who did not use intoxicants, did not smoke, had the least amount of meat in their diets and did not go to extremes in any respect. They have all been married, enjoyed their descendants and lived in a noble way.

They were wise and sparing in their actions. They were prudent, saving and carefully administering to their bodies just what they could handle. They never extended the body beyond what it could repair and rebuild, or beyond what it needed.

Because they were prudent and exercised wisdom, they never did anything that would cause troubles tomorrow, even though they could get by today. They lived as though they were going to do the same thing from day to day. They didn't do anything their bodies didn't want to do, and they followed the natural way with the same habits from day to day.

IT IS EXPERIENCE THAT HELPS US

The devitalized and denatured food that man has been eating for the past twenty-five years or more is now being fed to laboratory animals in experiments to determine the nutritive values of modern, processed foods; and these experiments are revealing that such devitalized foods produce disease in laboratory animals when fed on a constant diet of such foods. *What a Wonderful Discovery!* But this fact has been known by some for many years. Our body must have a right way of maintaining itself. It is for us to find the way we are meant to live, rather than try to live the way we would like to live.

Over a period of years I have seen health reappear by getting people to change their bad habits that create disease to good habits that create health. While many scientific facts can be proven by experiments on animals, I will say, that my work in dealing with human beings has proven to me that my theory and practice is right.

In the beginning of time there were no French cooks or graduate nurses. Where did our French dressing come from? Where did our cooked foods come from? Who got the idea of putting soda in our vegetables so that cooking would not alter their green color? Who put the cigarette in man's mouth? Who concocted our "scientific dope" to give us life, vigor and health?

With all of man's knowledge, I do not think he will ever know how much of the apple actually goes into the making of the heart or the function of it, or how much colloidal movement or action is put into our vital chemical elements. What is the need of the body? Who knows? It is this colloidal action that is found in our live foods and missing in our dead foods that makes for life or death in our bodies.

Very little has been done to try and create good health, or to try and prolong life, or to see how healthy people get along with each other. A few experiments have been worked out to create a healthy body. One of these was in seeing how little of the right food is necessary for a person to keep in good health.

Comaro lived over a hundred years. Seven different doctors had given him up to die at the age of forty. By cutting down his diet to such an extent that he did not make his body use more than just what food was necessary to get along on, he outlived these doctors.

Most of us fill our bodies with so much food we cannot take care of it, and I believe this habit amounts to a "killing process". This was proven in a little health experiment by a doctor at Cornell University. He had two controls of rats—he gave one group all the food they wished and gave the other group only half the amount of food the others ate. He found the rats that had half-rations lived twice as long. This truly is something for us humans to consider.

Thomas Edison said, "I keep my health by dieting. People gorge themselves with rich foods, use up their time, ruin their digestion and poison themselves. If the doctors would prescribe dieting instead of drugs, the ailments of normal man would disappear. Half the people are food drunk all the time. Dieting is my secret of health."

Calcium and Inheritance

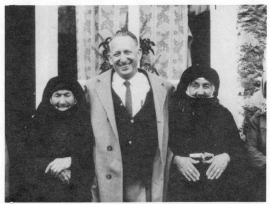

In Armenia we met this 127-year-old woman with her 85-year-old daughter.

The elderly people had lived in their particular region for their entire lives. Their families had lived there for many centuries and they became acclimated to the climate, to the foods. The body molded to this so much that it didn't have to start off in another direction and rebuild another type of body. Most of the inherited weaknesses had been lived out.

They didn't use an extreme amount of sugars or sweets or desserts. They didn't have an extreme amount of pressure, company, problems, troubles, civilization. They had lived a very even life and the genes had been developed in their bodies over a period of years. They had built bodies to withstand the elements.

People who have lived in sunshine valleys in the past, when brought to a high altitude cannot acclimate and this brings on disease. The body cannot react well to a lack of sunshine if it has been used to it in the past.

For those born at the ocean, born of people who for centuries lived at the ocean, it is difficult to go to the high altitudes, acclimate, and live a long time in just one generation. It takes inheritance through many centuries to produce a good body to live the long life.

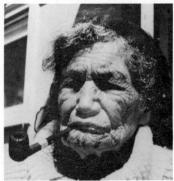

Maori from New Zealand, 123 years of age. While we found elderly people who had habits of which we did not approve, they still lived most of the Keys.

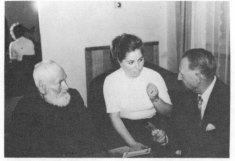

Most of the Keys are in their environment for centuries. Because of this, their genes provided bodies to live this long life. This is Mr. Gasanov of Russia at 153 years of age during our visit with him at a Baku T.V. Station.

Note the pigeon chests of the De Colorado Indians, caused by a lack of calcium. This can be caused either by a leached-out soil or a poor physical inheritance. The hair is plastered with achiota berries, giving a cap-like effect.

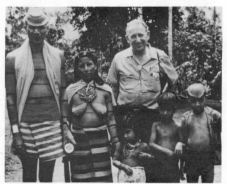

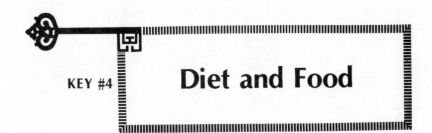

Diet and Food

Diet and foods are probably the most important Key. All of the old people lived on natural foods. They lived on berries, seeds, sprouts, greens, right from the field. Their foods were very simple. They didn't pay any attention to combinations. They brought out what is stated in the definition of good health, from the Teutonic, which is that health is our salvation.

This health comes when the foods are natural, pure, and whole. This is the foundation of their diet. When I asked them about their foods, they didn't know a person was supposed to have a diet. They didn't know a person lived on anything but what came out of the fields. They believed that what they grew they should eat. They followed the seasons.

This is something man in the city has confused. He has citrus fruits in the winter time. They are a summer fruit. It is an eliminating fruit, it's a reducing food. He is having tropical fruit in the north. He is not following the seasons and not harvesting or planting according to God's plan. These people did that.

There is one thing I have noticed. All long-life people live where grapes grow. Wherever grapes are grown it is possible to live a long life. Many factors go along to make a long life when we live in the grape country. There are many foods I believe were important in keeping these men in good health and living a long life.

I feel that cabbage is one of the most important of all, and especially with the Russians. We saw, coming into Moscow every morning, hundreds and hundreds of trucks and trailers loaded down with cabbage. Cabbage has the heating element, sulphur, for the body. It gave them the energy to resist the cold and the winter. It is one of their fine foods. The outside leaves are high in chlorophyll.

In the Hunza valley, 60% of the foods they were eating were fruits and vegetables grown in the sunshine. I call them sunshine foods because they control the calcium in the body. In order to have a long life you need foods with a lot of calcium. The black soil always had a lot of calcium in it. The glacial waters coming into the Hunza valley brought the silt and the minerals from the mountainside. This is what mineralized the terraces and gave the soil its proper mineral balance, bringing to the foods the elements to keep these people well.

One of the things we saw in these elderly people is that they had a lot of sodium in their diet. Sodium is a youth element. One of the things highest in sodium is whey. Whenever they took one of the dominant foods in their diet, which is clabbered milk, there was always a whey left over. Whey has the highest sodium content of any food. They used it as a drink and always gave it to the old men. This is the one element that kept their joints active, pliable, limber. It is one of the greatest deterrents to arthritis. There were never any stiff joints or arthritis in any of the old men I met. Another food high in sodium, to take care of their joints, was boiled joints and bones from the lamb. This also is a high sodium-content food.

These people did not use a lot of cow milk, but rather used goat's milk and sheep's milk, which is much higher in sodium and fluorine; and fluorine in combination with calcium gives long-life bones and a long-life body. Fluorine gives a hardness to the teeth and a hard structure to the outside of the bones. This is a long-life principle.

These elderly people used foods we don't even think of too much, from a long life standpoint. One of them is garlic. They used this to keep away colds. They used it to keep healthy and well. They used comfrey. They wrapped garlic in comfrey leaves, dried it, put it away, and made soup out of it in the winter time, which I think is a wonderful suggestion in this country for those who want to build up a good resistance and keep away from the catarrhal problems that usually accompany cold winter months.

They took rose hips and made a tea out of it. They used the surrounding herbs, camomile and the surrounding leaves from the bushes to make teas. This way they were able to prevent many sicknesses we are prone to because we do not use the herbs from the field.

The elderly people had a plentiful amount of protein in

their diet. I have never been too keen about having too much protein in the diet; in fact, I thought it was overdone years ago and I felt protein wasn't necessary. But, when you visit the little country of Helaconia where the average person only lives to 30, you find that they have increased this to 45 years of age by just adding a protein to their meals. Before they were living on raw sugar, raw corn and cornmeal. Now they have added soy milk powder, and 60% of the combination of raw sugar and cornmeal they were having is now made up of soy milk powder. To increase their life span by just adding a little protein is something to think about.

The Health Minister of India says that 86% of the diet served the Indian people is lacking protein; and coincidentally, India has one of the lowest life spans in the world. The average person, when I first went to India 35 years ago, was 21 years of age. Today the life span is running from 31 to 35 years of age. It still is very low, but they are also still low in protein.

Among these elderly people I met, I found very few vegetarians. We find that they did have a little meat. It was eaten sparingly, two or three times a week. Then we found they had other proteins, as in the Hunza valley where they used the apricot kernel, which is practically the same as the almond in its protein value. They were using walnuts, almonds and the clabber milk. They were having the clabber milk, which is a very high protein food, two times a day. I feel these suggestions from the elderly people were responsible for part of their long life.

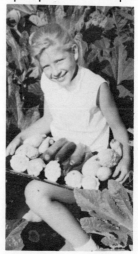

Hidden Valley Health Ranch

Foods throughout the world should be used in their natural state. But I am sure what man does to these foods as they come to his kitchen determines whether he has a healthy long life or not.

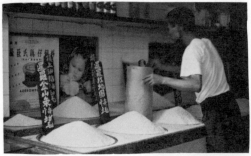

China

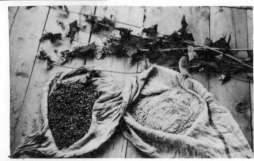

Hunza

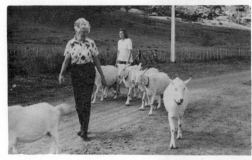

New Zealand

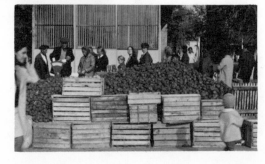

Russia

New Zealand

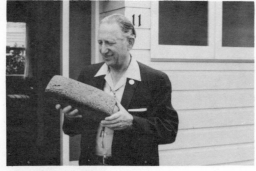

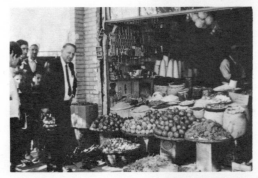

Iran

Iran

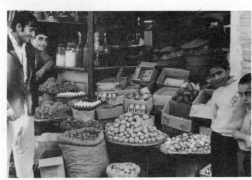

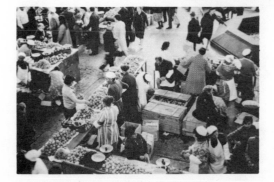

Armenia

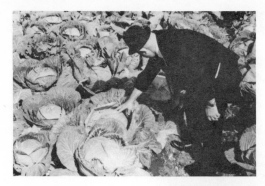

Armenia

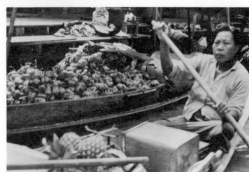

Thailand

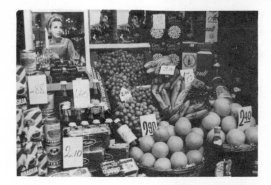

Finland

South Sea coconuts.

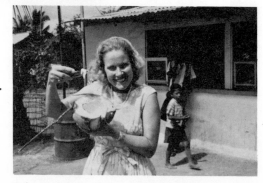

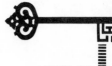

KEY #5

Circulation

Circulation is important because we must keep the blood flowing. There are three rules in keeping a good body: First, good blood, and that comes from good food, sunshine, water, etc. It is very important to have rest, the second rule, and to be able to recuperate when we are not tired. Rest doesn't always mean just going to bed; it could be rest from things that disturb you. But the third and most important thing is circulation. We must move the blood into parts of our body where we need regeneration and where regeneration must take place.

These people in there working don't have electric light buttons at shoulder height so they don't have to bend over. They are always bending, moving, reaching, stretching, lifting, pulling, pushing; the whole body is developed in the work they have. Too many of us live a sedentary life; we sit, we are executives, we drive, and we find that many of our heart troubles are developed because of our constant driving in automobiles.

We can carry milk cans up two or three flights of stairs. We can do this by carrying one at a time, that is, loaded.

We become one-sided in some of our playing and our exhibitions, such as in fencing. We do not have an even distribution of exercising as in the work of these old people. In keeping the circulation good, we keep the joints limber. Many of us do not use our bodies enough in order to have limber joints.

BARE FEET
[An article from the Auckland Star,
Monday, November 25, 1973]
This may interest correspondents who think that going about barefoot is unhygienic. Many years ago, in early childhood, a member of our family had a severe attack of

pleurisy, and every winter afterwards he suffered badly from croup. Then we moved to another district, which meant another doctor.

A fine old "family doctor", his advice shocked our mother. He said, "Send him to school barefoot during the winter, and when he plays outside the house in winter let him play barefoot. Let the other children do the same. It's from damp or wet socks and shoes a child catches cold— never from bare feet." Despite anxiety about it, our mother followed his advice, and there was never any more croup from that time onward. In later years another doctor told us that, when feeling tired, one of the best things to do is to go outside and walk on the lawn barefoot—even when the grass is wet. In dry weather it is a very good thing to lie down on the grass, so that as much of the body as possible comes in contact with the earth, because all of the body is thus refreshed. It need be done for just a few minutes. Going barefoot, therefore, is nothing to worry about. It may not look "dressy," but it's healthy.

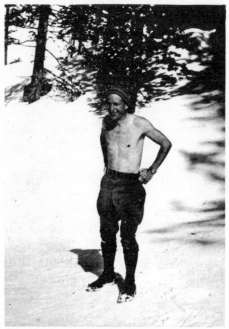

I was interested in improving my circulation, and snow baths are one way of doing it. I took these snow baths to develop a good circulation in my body. I heard about Father Kneippe curing his own lung ailment when he was in his 20's by walking in the snow.

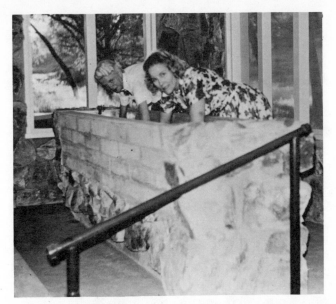

A good circulation was found in all elderly people, and an inactive flow of blood will shorten a person's life.

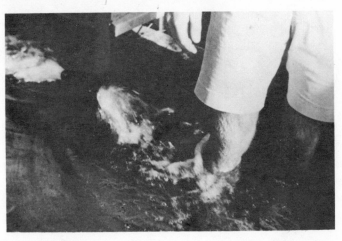

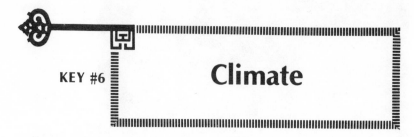

KEY #6   Climate

INCLUDING ALTITUDE AND AIR

Climate, altitude and air are three of the most important factors in gaining health and in maintaining it. Where all three factors are correctly present, it is a salubrious environment for man's heartbeat, his elimination and an elevated blood count. From this one can deduce that there is a proper place in which to live that is healthful for us.

The importance of these three factors requires that we write at greater length about them elsewhere in this book.

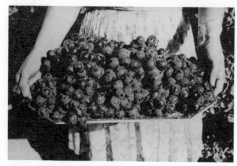

The oldest people in the world always live in a place where grapes are grown.

The thermal cure of Switzerland helps to bring people to a balance that is necessary for their health.

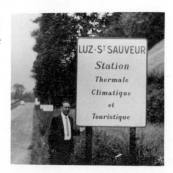

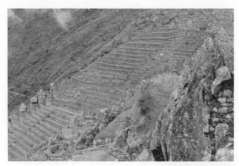

The mountain tops at Machu Pacchu, South America, are above the sultry jungle life below.

Hunza terraces at 6,000 to 7,000 feet.

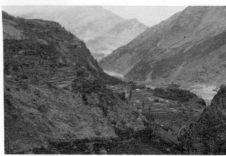

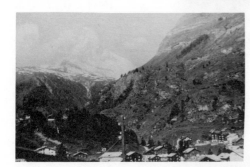

The altitude of the Swiss mountains quickens the thyroid gland and produces a higher blood count.

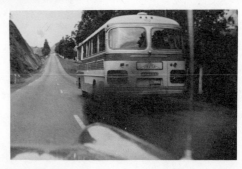

Pure air is a necessity and rarefied air in the mountains seems to be where the old men live—not where exhaust fumes come from trucks and cars like this.

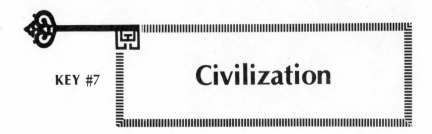

KEY #7

Civilization

SOCIETY

We have a very resentful and permissive society these days. We have a society that allows people to do almost anything—to reject, discard, and to violate anything that does not suit one's individual fancy. We no longer have set up a society to do what is right but rather we do "who" is right.

It is difficult to uptalk a person these days, because everyone seems to have taken on an individual pattern of living that few can follow. Everyone seems to be but for himself. Society has become resentful and even selfish.

We have no longer followed the old precept of "Love ye one another"; and "What ye have done unto the least of these, ye do unto Me also."

We are closer than ever from a travel standpoint and communication standpoint; yet we are further apart in walking the united way. Man will never be agreed until he learns how to walk together.

One person could have a sad experience and measure all of society by that experience. Somebody is satisfied with coffee and donuts, and thinks all of society should follow that.

The average person has lost his tact today and his tolerance. Suzy hates Peter. Peter hates Suzy, and then they both hate war.

The differences we have in our food routine and our treatment routine has brought on a lot of animosity and ill feelings. There are many people who know that you can't take flour and water, add vitamins, and make a good product. But we have been taught today to sell the crunch, the pop, or the sizzle.

You are killing us, man! Much of the food problems today should be investigated to see if they are natural, pure and whole. I am sure that while many know this is a necessary part of good living, probably 90 % of the people would reject it. They need teaching. They need understanding. They need knowledge, and above all they need enlightenment and wisdom.

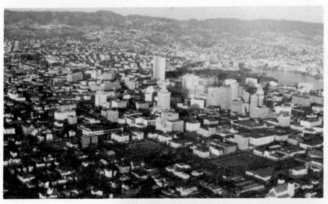

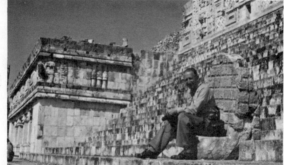

City life can kill us.

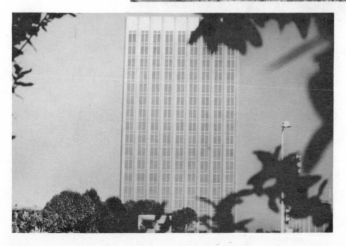

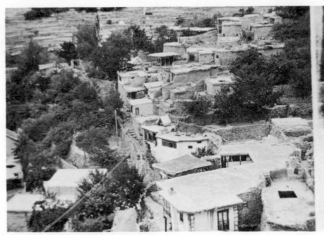

Hunza buildings are simple, yet those who live within them live a longer life.

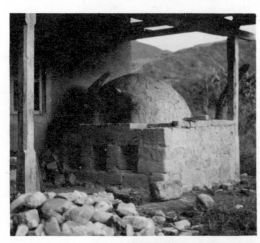

Cooking foods is a long way from the Garden of Eden.

You can still find markets with natural foods in the cities. This is Farmer's Market in Los Angeles.

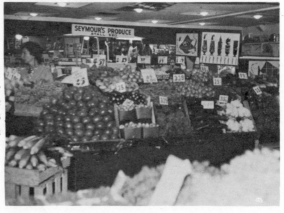

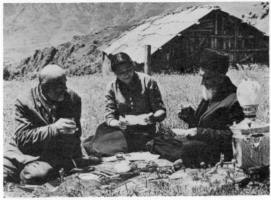

Russian scene with
Shirali Mislimov
[167 years of age].

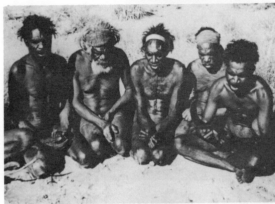

Aborigines in
Australia.

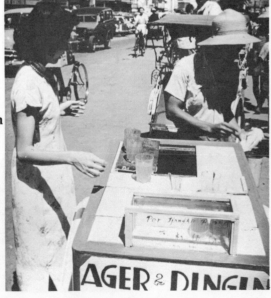

Soft drink wagon in
Djakarta.

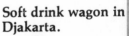

149

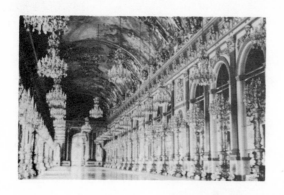

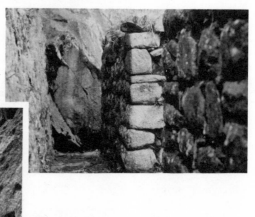

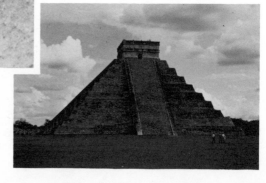

Man has gone a long way from the dance halls of Germany to the simple architecture and living habits of our past cultures.

Transportation.

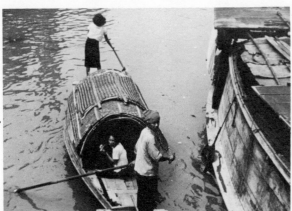

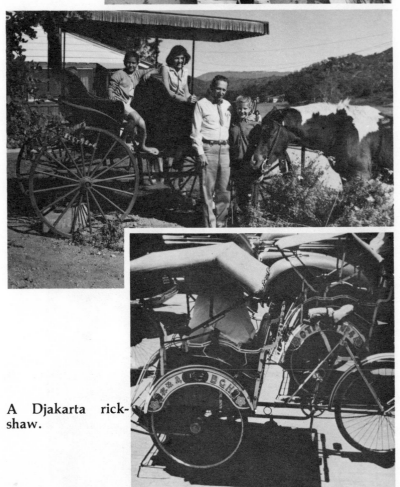

A Djakarta rickshaw.

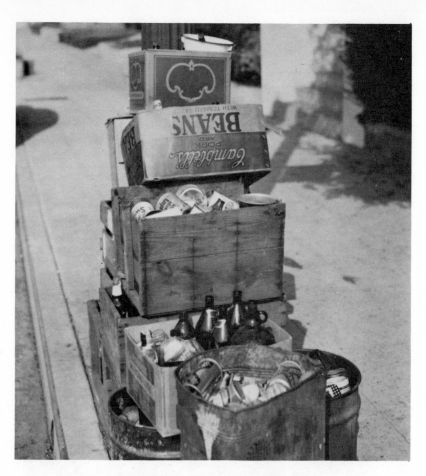

Civilized foods can kill you.

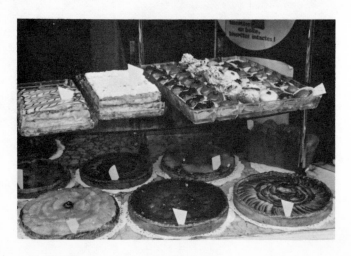

Activity and Retirement

RETIRING

All the old men I met were thankful to be able to work. Work is the greatest pleasure we have in our lives. When I talk to patients, the unable and the ailing, they are all heading for one thing: to get back to work.

It is a blessing to be able to work. To be capable of activity on a job is the greatest blessing we have. Many people fight work today, but we should be thankful we can work.

All of these old men are working. If you want to see them, they are out in the field working. A man, 153 years

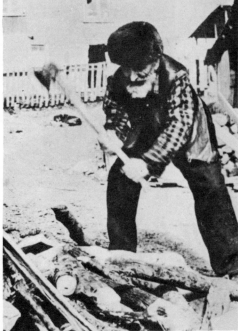

Mislimov is shown cutting wood at the age of 165.

of age, came riding in on horseback. The average man here, at the age of 60, can't even get on a horse anymore.

You have to have this idea of retiring at 60 taken out of your consciousness. (I have seen files of retired men in companies where at the age of 60 they were considered no good anymore and were being put out to pasture.) Man considers this as something natural in this country. We find the average man dies five years after he has retired.

So what do you do? You retire to death! Not to life! Most people think they can do with a few hundred dollars a month. It is the greatest thing in the world to be able to work and to be in good health.

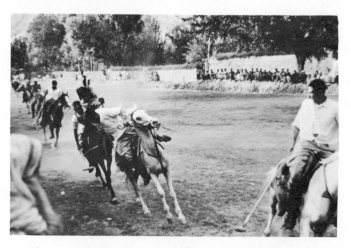

The world champion Gilgit polo team [Hunza].

These Mexican dancers continue for 7 days and nights.

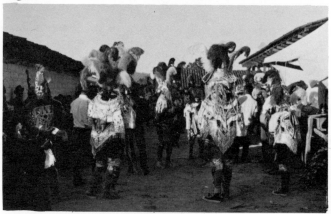

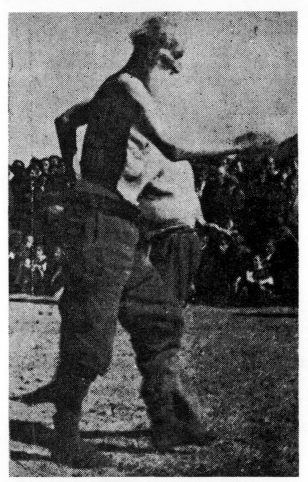

November 13, 1969 TURKEY

The contest of the oldest wrestlers in Turkey took place in the town of Resadiyie, where a surprise event occurred.

This gathering included over 180 of these men. They oiled their bodies, Turkish sytle, as is the custom at national events and weddings.

During the wrestling event there is always village music consisting of a "Davull" (a big parade drum covered with goat skin to give a full and strong ring) and the Zurna, resembling the Chinese clarinet, playing the customary tune of the well-known "Cezayir".

This theme is traditional for national events, weddings, and before an attack on an enemy in the war.

During the festivities, the oldest man, 110 years old, who was only a spectator, became so stimulated by the thump of the drum and music that he ran to the oil (kazan) bucket, stripped, put on his "kisbet" (oiled wrestling breaches) and rushed into the middle of the ring and asked if anyone would like to challenge him.

His name was Dursun Coban, 110 years old, from the town of Kirkpinar and he called for a match!

A very well-known head wrestler, named Hasan Ozturk, answered his challenge. Both men oiled and with the same traditional rules began to wrestle.

After a short bout, on the very first fall, the 110-year-old Dursun Coban threw his 70-year-old opponent out of the ring. Dursun Coban, 40 years older, maintained his title.

To play the game of life, you have to be active, on the move, with a good limber body.

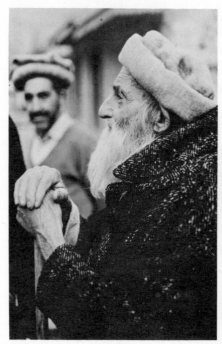

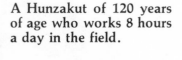

A Hunzakut of 120 years of age who works 8 hours a day in the field.

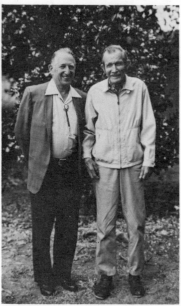

Dave Powers at the age of 82 still has walking records that remain unbroken.

To play the game of life, you have to be active, on the move, with a good limber body.

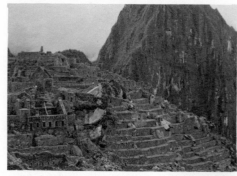

The past civilization of Machu Picchu, was built on the top of a mountain [South America].

Grass and sand walking for active circulation.

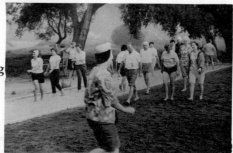

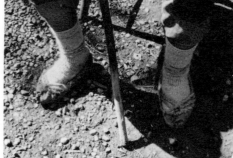

Soft shoes for walking on uneven ground keeps leg muscles in good tone.

New Mexican Indian runner.

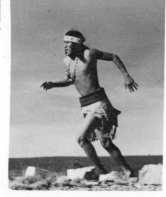

Keep the Aging Active, Say Experts

Society makes a mistake in expecting persons to greatly reduce their physical and mental activity as they grow older, according to experts today at the Western Gerontological Society meeting here.

"Older people should not be permitted to rest more and more and more," Dr. Steven M. Horvath, director of the Institute of Environmental Stress at the University of California, Santa Barbara, told an audience of some 900 persons at the Los Angeles Hilton.

"If you use it, fine; if you don't use it, it just goes to pieces," Horvath said, noting that many of the physical changes associated with aging are related to disuse.

A decline in the bodily health is "facilitated by a tendency to force older people to rest," Horvath said, noting that all age groups today are less active than their counterparts in the 1930s.

Desert retirement communities may pose a problem to older persons, he said.

He said older persons take up to three times longer to adapt to heat as do young persons and "more old people die in heat spells than do young people."

The intelligence of older persons is widely underestimated, said Dr. Carl Eisdorfer, chairman of the Department of Psychiatry at the University of Washington School of Medicine.

He said intelligence levels remain relatively stable throughout a person's life until two or three years before death, but that older persons tend to withdraw from active learning.

"It's not that they can't do it, but that they won't," said Eisdorfer, adding, "What's worse than that is that the culture reinforces that pattern."

Lowered performance on intelligence tests by older persons is the result of impaired health, social isolation, economic level, limited education and lower motivation, rather than a decline in ability, said Eisdorfer.

Sponsored by the University of Southern California Gerontology Center, the three-day session is titled "Making the Knowledge Explosion Work for the Elderly" and will conclude tomorrow.

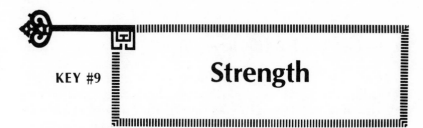

KEY #9

Strength

In the Psalms they say that our years will be three-score and ten; but, if we should be strong, they may be four-score. I believe this may be so, for as we look to the elderly people we see they are strong people. They have lived in communities and countries where it took a lot of strength to move aside rocks to make roads. Stones were used to build houses; dams and waterways were erected. they lived in the hills where it took a lot of strength to walk and to accomplish deeds.

This strength, I am convinced, is what gave them their added years. Bernarr McFadden said, "Keep your muscles in good order, because every activity in your body is dependent upon the muscles you have."

When you walk, you move the blood around; when you sit there is very little activity. When you work, muscles are developed. When you play games, muscles are developed. Strength is one of the notable qualities men were admired for in the past.

Strength is what conquers from a physical standpoint. I never recognized the greatness of this until I traveled to Turkey. I went to the northern part of Greece and Macedonia and saw where Alexander the Great traveled east through Turkey, picking up an army of 30,000 men and conquering various places by just sheer strength. His army and activities brought him through Persia unconquered because of their strength.

In Turkey we find some of the oldest and strongest men in the world. The champion of their wrestling team in Turkey is 75 years old.

. I saw an old man carying a piano on his back for 15 blocks. He was 75 years old! Strength is a great thing; in fact, a man must have his strength when he marries because this is an ideal to the wife and family. Strength is indicative of a good glandular and a good sexual system.

It was through strength that man was able to conquer nature with the resistance to overcome and dam up the walls of a flooding river. This was their ideal that they had to overcome nature. When you are close to the soil, close to nature, you have to have strength to battle the elements.

It is only the strong who survive. Nature is not interested in the weak; she eliminates the weak and it is the fit who survive. Strength was one of the inherent qualities brought to the Hunza Valley. It was Alexander the Great who brought this army of strength to the Hunza River where he died. But, six of his officers left his army, went up through Afghanistan down into the Hunza Valley to establish themselves with their Persian wives in the Valley we consider Shangri-La today.

In one section of Turkey strength is demonstrated by the amount of weight people can carry on their backs.

The Bible says that our life should be threescore and ten, but if we have strength, our life will be fourscore.

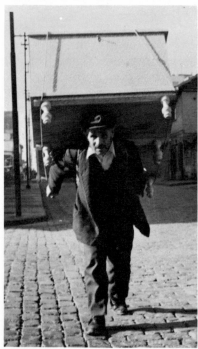 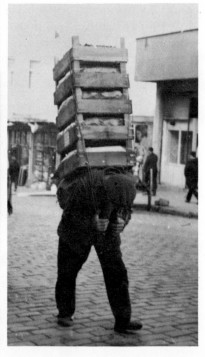

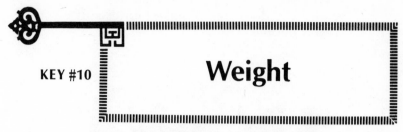

Weight

This is another key. It has been said, many times, the bigger the waistline, the smaller the lifeline. Those people who have lived the longest are those who are 16 lbs. underweight according to insurance statistics. In checking with all of these old people, none of them have a body much heavier than they had when they were 20 years of age.

BEING OVERWEIGHT IS SERIOUS

Weight reduction is one of the biggest problems of people in this country today.

We find that overweight is considered the Number One killer, surpassing deaths attributed to cancer, heart conditions, diabetes, and alcoholism. The longer the waistline, the shorter the lifeline. Scientific research is proving that overweight actually is a disease. When a person has overweight to contend with, he is dealing with a malfunction of the vital organs in his body. This can affect the heart, the kidneys, and the digestive organs. It can be the cause of many troubles and also be a symptom of many glandular disturbances. It is a very uncomfortable condition of the flesh, causing more disturbances through pressure symptoms than anything else—pressure against the kidneys, the heart, and various organs. By interfering with the proper blood and nerve supply, pressures can produce an anemic condition through impaired blood circulation, so that degeneration may set in. Water collects in the tissues, affecting the increase in body weight.

In developing this flabby flesh, persons usually develop a "flabby" will power. Those who have good muscular tone invariably have greater power to make decisions.

Whatever may be the cause, resolve now to begin to correct it.

Unjust Desserts

Now tempt me with no sight or whiff
Of cake or pie, lest I be grabby.
Ah, why does starch make fabrics stiff
And people flabby?

by Janet Merchant

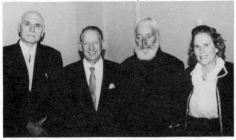

This is Peter Maloff, myself, Mr. Gasanov and Marie in Baku, Russia. One of the main Keys is that the elderly maintained the same weight they had between the ages of 20 and 30 during their later years.

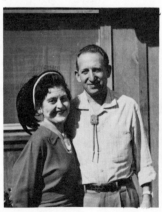 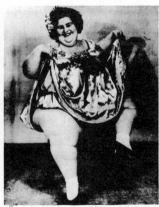

The lady in the photo weighed well over 500 lbs., but with sensible dieting she reduced down to 110 lbs. The diet she used was very much like the one that the elderly people used throughout the world. In reduction of weight, many other diseases have diminished, namely: high blood pressure, kidney disturbances, heart pressure, cholesterol, fatigue and short windedness. A good fit body was developed by eating the proper foods and getting proper exercise. It is very important to prevent disease and to keep our weight balanced all of our lives.

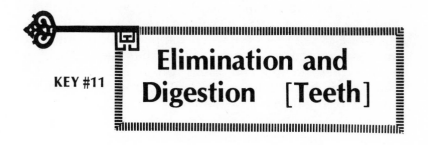

Elimination and Digestion [Teeth]

Digestion begins in the mouth. That first morsel of food is broken down by the teeth and mastication begins. This is where the proper amount of saliva is necessary, and of course the proper teeth are required to begin digestion.

One thing we noticed with the elderly people is that most of them have all of their teeth and that they are good teeth. They have no problems in chewing their foods. They chew rough foods and their jaws are strong. This brings a lot of blood to the gums and teeth by the fact that they chew a lot of raw foods and hard foods such as nuts, seeds, grains, etc.

By demonstrating the relationships between the teeth and the functions of the body, we realize that if the food isn't prepared properly for the stomach and intestinal tract we can begin various conditions such as indigestion, ulcers, colitis, etc.

We have found through experiments with cows that when the teeth in elderly cows were repaired, their digestion was improved so much that they were able to give almost double the amount of milk.

It takes the proper amount of enzymes and hydrochloric acids to break down the proteins in the stomach and intestinal tract. We find that hospital reports show that people over the age of 50 have a lack of hydrochloric acid. They do not digest proteins properly. As you may know, proteins are very important for carrying on the life processes in the body. If the stomach does not have the necessary amount of hydrochloric acid, we have to eat foods that have been prepared so they are easy to digest, easy to assimilate and can be readily absorbed when they do get to the intestinal tract.

I find that the old men were using koumas, clabbered milk, yogurt and forms of soured, clabbered milk. I believe one of the first things that happens to any milk product when it reaches the stomach is that the hydrochloric acid curdles the milk and brings it to the soured, or clabbered state. But if there is a lack of hydrochloric acid, this process of digestion is weakened.

The elderly men use a good deal of this clabbered milk which is unheated and just as nature meant for them to have it. In this way, I feel they are able to get the proper amount of protein in an easily digestible form and in the most natural way it can be brought to the body.

This is one of the secrets why the Bulgarians have more people over 100 years of age, according to their population, than any other country in the world. They used a buttermilk—they used an acidophilus milk—and we find that this particular bacteria grew at a certain altitude and in a certain climate.

This friendly bacteria for the intestinal tract is explained so well by Metchnikoff. He told us how the intestinal tract should be toxic-free and have no infections for the body to absorb.

The Bulgarians had the least amount of toxemia, had the least amount of sickness developing, because they had none of these low-grade infections.

We need to have the proper amount of hydrochloric acid or it will seriously interfere with gastric digestion, and putrefaction and intestinal disturbances in the large intestine will increase, thereby causing gas.

The lack of hydrochloric acid may be due to nervous disturbances or too much work. Yet again, when we see these old people, they were not suffering from either of these problems. We must remember that the secretion of this acid is more easily disturbed than that of pectin and other digestive enzymes.

In digestion we have to have the proper amount of saliva. This comes from a lymph flow in the body. The lymph glands are found in the parts of the body that we move most—along the neck, spine, lung structure, under the arm and groin; and their activities and motion have these lymph glands moving the lymph fluids along, developing a good secretion of the saliva.

Breathing always favors the saliva flow. This was well developed by walking in the hills and living in a balanced climate.

Digestion begins in the mouth and ends in the lungs. It goes on into the blood and lungs where the blood is oxygenized, which is the last and most important part of digestion.

Digestion is not strictly vegetative. It is more psychic than we know. If the vegus nerve is cut, digestion is impossible. If there is no gastric juice whatever, and no hydrochloric acid in the stomach, digestion is again impossible; and if one eats at such a time he will only suffer from indigestion, fermentation, or gas.

There are some types of people who have a stronger digestive ability than others. Constipation and intestinal stasis is the one thing where more money is made in the doctor's office than any other complaint. It is most universal and directly responsible for about 90 % of human ailments today.

The nicest thing I can say about the elderly people in taking care of the colon is that they were doing the right thing. They used certain types of whey to develop a bacteria and a certain acid-alkaline balance—a certain lactic balance. This only takes place when we have whey from cows that live and pasture at a certain altitude. I am convinced that the people who live at this altitude have a bacteria develop in their bowel with the milk that helps to give them their long life.

Elimination is very important. It's like bringing all the food into the kitchen and then finding that the garbage disposal doesn't work, or materials from the kitchen that have been left over are not taken out. The day comes when a mess accumulates in the kitchen.

One of the great things I can tell you is that with a lowered vital resistance we are prone to disease. It is very, very important to prevent disease, and we find that the more diseases we have, the more coughs, bronchial troubles, accumulations of catarrh that produce discharges through the ears, tonsils, or other organs of elimination which lowers the vital energy of the body, and in time, causes a short life.

It is very important to realize that we must take care of the intestinal tract. The elderly people with the proper exercises, such as bending over, pulling, pushing, hoeing, and working in the garden have kept the intestinal tract in good order.

There is one thing in their lives that is an important factor: they had no inhibitions in going to the bathroom. Whenever they need to go, they go, no matter where they are. They are not waiting till they reach the next town, they are not driving around and holding it, they are never too busy to have a bowel movement. When I asked all the elderly men if they had bowel movements every day, they said, "Why, of course, doesn't everybody?" They don't know what the rest of the world is doing. Laxatives, purgatives, enemas and colonics are the biggest business we have today in the healing arts.

FALSE LIVING—FALSE TEETH

One of my own recent experiences brought this home to me plainly. An eleven-year-old boy was sent in to me by another doctor and upon checking this boy, I found that he had a complete set of dentures! When we have to face the fact that a boy of eleven has to have dentures, it is time to start doing something about this horrible scourge! Every sincere and thinking medical man or healer today should be giving a great deal of his time and energy to this problem.

Another dentist sent a young chap in to our office; most of his teeth were gone. He was only 12 year old and we are showing a picture of his teeth. The dentist claimed he could not do anything with these teeth; that it was a body condition. What a shame to see these teeth, the beautiful pearls of the mouth, broken down when, after all, good food could be taking care of them.

EAT GREENS

We know that teeth are broken down and deteriorated when a person does not live right and follow a proper diet. In our diet, greens are most important as they control the calcium in the body. The Hunzas, who had such beautiful teeth and kept them until they died at over 100 years of age, followed a diet in which they ate a lot of greens and the tops of vegetables. We should eat more parsley, beet greens, watercress, spinach and the many different greens which we can get in salads daily. These will help to keep our teeth right.

Observe from the following statistics, published by the Register General of England, that no group has contributed more to the death rate from intestinal disease than doctors. On the other hand, those who have the least intestinal disorders are the agricultural laborers.

Physicians, surgeons .50
Inn keepers 45
Barristers, solicitors 44
Seamen 43
Clergymen, priests, ministers 34
Butchers 30
Carmen, carriers 28
Farmers 25
Gardeners 22
Railway guards, porters 20
Agricultural laborers 19
Average among all workers 28

As shown by the above statistics, the death rate of doctors is 31 points higher than that of the agricultural laborer, and 22 points higher than that of the average death rate of all other workers, who die of diseases of the digestive system.

A VISIT TO DR. GEORGE W. HEARD, A TEXAS DENTIST

We have just visited with Dr. George W. Heard in Hereford, Texas. For years they have been heralding Dr. Heard's account, his work, and his field of dentistry. He has written a lot about the teeth, and man's troubles with the teeth.

The thirty years that Dr. Heard has been a dentist in Hereford, Texas, he has not pulled out a single tooth from anyone who lived in that city. He claims that the food they ate, that the diet they lived on, and the particular community was responsible for the good teeth that these people had. He has written a book called 'Man Vs Toothache'. Thirty years as a dentist and never to have found a cavity in any of the teeth of the people who lived in his home town is certainly something to think about.

The last time I visited him he autographed one of his books which certainly is a tribute to the 'new day' thinking, especially when he writes that nutrition is the foundation of all good health. It was wonderful to see a man of 93 years of age carrying on the good work of demonstrating good health. He maintained that the plant life produced from a well-balanced soil contained the proper elements that were needed for health. He believes that so much of our food has been so tampered with today that it is the beginning of a good deal of our body troubles, and of course, it finally gets to the teeth. He showed us many pictures of teeth and how wonderful they were when the owner of them lived on good foods. He was a great believer of raw milk.

We cannot help but remember how Captain Cook when traveling through the South Seas saw his sailors lose activity and the power to lift and to carry on with their work when they lived on the civilized foods that they carried with them. He tells in his history and his diary about the South Sea Islanders who lost their many athletic abilities when they started living on the civilized foods that were brought to them.

Stephenson showed that the bones lost their natural function when the calcium had been taken from the civilized foods that were fed to them. It was Dr. Price that showed we could not have good teeth unless we were fed right, that as the body began to break down, the teeth would break down also, and that the teeth were an integral part of the body, and that calcium was one of the most important elements to have in our bodies.

This has been demonstrated in many experiments with animals. The bones, the structure of the body is dependent upon the element calcium for it is the knitter, it gives the power, the tone, the repair material that keeps our bodies alkaline. It is the element that is needed for long life and a good life.

Dr. Heard was most emphatic in his remarks that we must have the proper wheat and the proper flour in our diets otherwise this could be one of the most effective things in breaking down the structures. He was telling me how the bakery has to make bread according to his specifications, but found later they had changed the specifications so much that he refused to have his name on the wrapper. He was a stickler for the right thing as far as food was concerned. He changed over to raw food at 50 when he had been 'given up' during a serious illness. It was surprising to see him at the age of 93 in fairly good health. He said he had been in very good health since he was 50 when he changed to natural foods.

He told me that no one could be sick and would be sick by living on mostly raw food. He believed in raw milk especially. Dr. Heard's philosophy was found in just these few words, "The popular foods served today are disease-creating, and the diseases that attack us are of our own creation. Man has the power of choice; whatever he has, he has chosen." Any town can be a town without a toothache if the people choose it. Most dentists believe that taking too much citrus fruit is not good for the teeth and especially the lemon juice that many people are using. We are showing a picture here where lemon juice has been used for many years to wash the teeth which has caused the enamel to disintegrate.

It was Dr. Price that summed up his findings in his book on nutritional and physical degeneration. That manual is a must for every dentist who would understand the role that food and drink plays in building sound teeth. The evidence which he gathered in his exploration evidenced that what he set down in great detail, has led Dr. Price to conclude that the primitive man would be free of tooth decay and at the same time be free of the white man's diseases as long as he lived out of contact with modern civilization and its refined foods, but lived where he could obtain sea food.

It was Dr. Heard that said in his own findings in Deaf Smith County that beyond a shadow of a doubt, the white man himself right in the middle of his own civilization with no contact with the sea; that is, without sea foods, man can have perfect teeth as long as he lives. Dr. Price showed great interest in Dr. Heard's work in Hereford, Texas and even sent for some of the milk and cream from the Bonnie Brumley's farm in Deaf Smith County. He learned to work seeming magic with butterfat that was produced from the cows grazing on Mr. Brumley's green wheat. For example, when he fed that cream to an arthritis patient the arthritic pain disappeared for that time. But when Mr. Brumley would take his cows off green wheat, Dr. Price would immediately notice the difference in the type of cream he was getting. Dr. Price would write you have changed your feed' the last lot of cream you sent to me does not measure up to the usual standard. It is short on vitamins and various minerals which my patients require. It sure was strange to see how the doctor could tell the difference in his patients to this extent.

Dr. Price confided in Dr. Heard and said, "You Deaf Smith County soil contains an element which has not been named. This special element is very powerful when assimilated from this wheat and other plants; I call it Activator X." Much could be said about these experiments but as we read and go through the work on nutrition we will see that it is a very workable thing to keep the whole body well and alive and in good health if we keep eating good foods, no matter what organ is ailing.

Dentists never catch up with their work. For instance, New York City has approximately 9,000 dentists to take care of the mouths of its 8 million people, yet about 35 million tooth cavities are untreated. The teeth constitute less than one percent of the body whether we judge by bulk or weight. There are about 100,000 dentists in the United States, but the care of the rest of the body rests upon about 250,000 physicians.

THE TEETH

The human tooth is actually very similar to a fish scale. A shark's scale and a human tooth correspond completely in their basic structure.

A tooth is a projection of the skin which has entered into an intimate union with the skeleton, in particular with the jaw, so as to obtain support. The part situated within the socket of the jaw is known as the root, the portion projecting beyond the gums is the crown, and the portion between these is called the neck.

In the root canal at the base of the root is an entrance for blood, lymph vessels and nerves. The principal mass of the tooth is composed of a bony substance known as dentine. On its outer surface the crown of the tooth is covered with enamel, as a finger by a thimble. The enamel has no nerves or blood vessels and is the hardest, most compact tissue of the entire body.

Chemically it consists of phosphate of lime, fluoride of calcium, carbonate of lime, phosphate of magnesium, as well as traces of other salts.

At birth a human infant is without teeth. After six

months, the first teeth appear in the center of the lower jaw, and in the course of about two years, a total of 20 teeth appear. These are known as milk teeth. Beneath these rest a second series of teeth (thirty-two) that begin to come out at about six years of age when the child begins to lose his first set. By the age of 21, all of the 32 permanent teeth have usually come into the mouth, with occasional exceptions of the third molars or wisdom teeth.

The most frequent dental disease is dental decay or caries. When a defect appears in the enamel, the bacteria present in the mouth wander into this break in the enamel and set to work destroying the dentine.

The basic cause of tooth decay is a diet dificient in calcium, or a diet containing an excess of concentrated carbohydrates which indirectly causes the calcium level in the blood to be lowered.

AMERICA'S DIETARY DIFICIENCIES SHOW UP IN ITS CITIZEN'S TEETH

The problem of tooth decay is one of the major problems of the dental and medical professions today, to say nothing of the expense that must be added on to the family budget to take care of the family's deteriorating teeth. A recent survey by the Public Health Service shows that more than 21 million Americans have lost all their teeth.

There are innumerable research programs being conducted in laboratories all over the world with just one idea in mind: "The prevention of tooth decay." Most of these research programs have recognized that the most glaring fact discovered to date is that this decay is caused from faulty diets and nutritional deficiencies.

Dr. Michael J. Walsh, director of clinical nutrition courses at the University of California Dental Extension in San Francisco says: "Americans are waterlogged and are suffering from dietary deficiencies—but don't know it. What the public mind looks upon as three square meals a day is likely to be a starvation diet and one that will decay the toughest tooth."

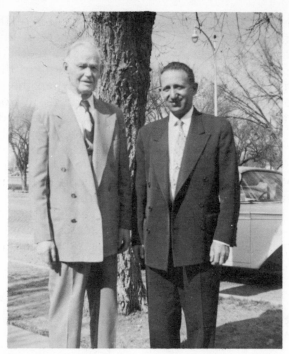

Dr. George W. Heard, a dentist, and I discussing the subject of teeth in Hereford, Texas.

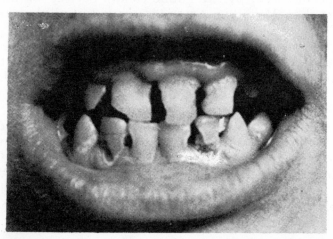

A dentist sent this twelve-year-old boy to me because his tooth decay was coming from an unbalanced diet lacking the proper chemical elements.

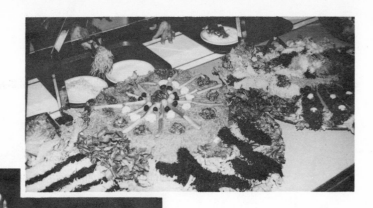

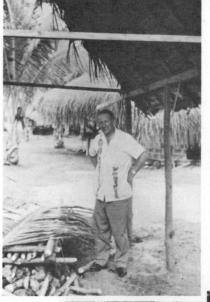

We begin digestion with our teeth and then make sure we have the proper foods. Customs around the world are all different. Food preparations are all different. I am sure the more we get away from natural foods the shorter is our life.

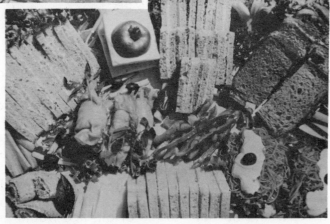

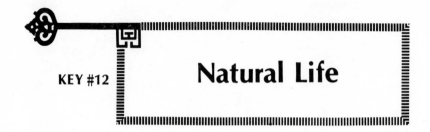

Natural Life

Wherever the old men lived, you found people living the natural life style. They lived in homes built by materials in the surrounding countryside. They lived an outdoor life and exercised; they lived by the sweat of their brow. They were happy.

They believed in having enough for everyone in their community, they helped one another; they shared; they had a lovely philosophy. We saw no greed among these people. It seems like there was enough for everybody. They followed the creed that there isn't enough for those in greed, but there is enough for those in need.

Their water was natural; foods were natural. They lived in pure mountain air, in a good climate, at a good altitude.

Civilization is coming upon these people and it is destroying the lovely features we find among them that make for a natural way of living.

NATURE IS JUST

Do we realize that if we left our beautiful homes for Nature to take care of, they would not last very long? Nature, the same as little boys, goes along to throw rocks and break windows; the paint wears thin; the roof requires care; the plumbing needs repairs. We must continue strengthening our house against the heat and cold. Even though it seems cruel and harsh, Nature is just. It treats all of us alike, whether we dwell in a palace or a shack. To benefit from Nature, we must learn to cooperate with her. If we would do that, to die of old age would be impossible. By not cooperating with Nature we kill ourselves with our own bad habits. Our lack of education in the matter of nutrition helps in this. It is said that it's not what you eat that kills you; it is sometimes what you did NOT eat that kills you. We can starve, abuse and over-use through lack of knowledge.

Think of the noisy civilization in which we live, with its heavy traffic, loud inharmonious sounds and personal problems which cause tension, all of which tend to shorten our lives. However, we are dying from a lack of education in nutrition more than anything else. When we think about prolonging our life, we must first put our mind in order. We will have to start with the entire person and then specialize so we will finally be able to know what is in the cell structure down to the fingernails. We must learn with a light heart and look to Godly ways.

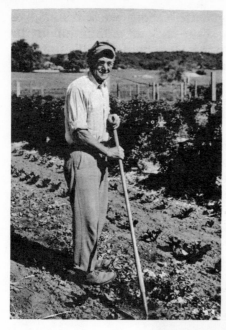

The man with a hoe is the man close to the soil. He keeps himself well by living the natural life.

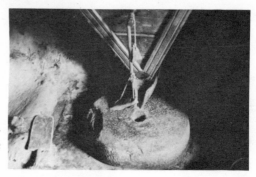

Stone grinding; a natural way to prepare flour.

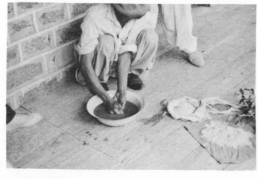

Extracting the oils from the apricot. The Hunzas use everything in the apricot; the fruit, kernal and the oils.

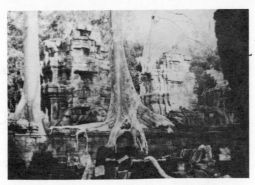

In the jungles of Cambodia lies Ankor Wat. When man does not work with nature; nature wins in the end. The roots of the trees have broken down the temples man built in the past.

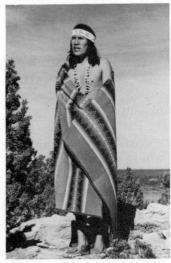

The Indian led a hard life but a colorful one.

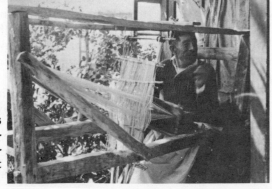

Keeping the fingers busy, the mind active and at a pleasant tempo is part of the natural life.

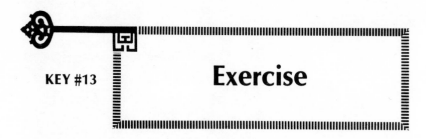

KEY #13

Exercise

Food alone will never make a person well. I'm convinced we could think well, but if we don't exercise, we will lose the use of our muscles. We lose the use of our bodies without exercise. Exercise is very, very important.

I saw a great scene unfolding, especially with the elderly people, when I noticed that the women do not live as long as the men. I am convinced it is because the men do not retire like the women do. The men constantly work, and their work is one where they use their leg muscles. They are constantly working with their sheep. They are walking on uneven ground all day. They are developing leg muscles for good circulation. Dr. Paul Dudley White, Eisenhower's physician, said, "Man dies from his feet up." Most sick people have cold feet where the circulation is poor. This is a sign that the extremities do not get enough proper circulation. The most important extremity is our head. I never found any senile, elderly people on my visits. I don't think senility allows us to grow old. But to keep away from senility we have to have a good circulation, and this good circulation is developed in the legs.

As we go through these Keys, as far as treatments are concerned, you will find that taking care of the legs is most important. One of the ways of doing this is found in Worishoven, Germany where they use the cold leg baths by walking in cold water, and then walking in the grass afterwards. If you just experiment enough with you own arms, you can see when you hold your arm very tightly with your hand, and wiggle your hand and fingers, all the muscles will move in your arm. But if you keep your arm moving back and forth, and your hand does not move, the hand muscles do not contract and move the muscles in the arm. In this way you will see and compare it to the structure of the legs. You have to walk barefooted in order

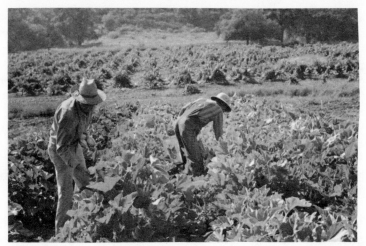
Working in the garden is one way of keeping the body well. Most of the people who have worked in the gardens here at Hidden Valley Health Ranch have improved in their health.

to have good circulation in the legs.

All the old men I visited had soft-soled shoes. They walked on uneven surfaces so all the small muscles of the legs were developed well and could keep that venous blood that needs to go back to the liver, circulating. It keeps it going uphill. We have to have strong legs and a strong muscle structure in order to get that blood going back up into the body to be oxygenated through the lung structure again. Arterial blood has a lot of oxygen in it. Venous blood, or the blood that is in the veins in our legs, needs more oxygen. It must have good muscle structure to move it out of the legs so it comes back a good red blood again with nourishment, with proper oxygen, so those legs are kept in good condition.

When the feet are cold, arthritis can settle in, calcium can come out of solution, corns develop, bunions develop; but it is in the extremities where we can usually look for our troubles. The feet can be a good barometer to your health. You can watch your toenails, the bony structure, the ligament structure. A person who has bad feet usually has some condition in another part of the body dependent upon the good condition of those feet, such as curvature of the spine or muscle tension. When a person can't walk and run properly, it affects the whole body.

One of the laws is to keep walking and you see this happening so much with these people that they must keep their bodies strong and healthy. They do this by physical activity. The women come inside of the house after age 80 or 85. The men are still working in the garden. Those men I met at 150, 153 years of age; there was no retirement. So keep walking, don't retire. Keep your body moving. I believe it is one of the greatest of the world Keys. Never retire. Keep your body active and keep it strong.

SECRET OF LONGEVITY

A prominent San Jose pioneer was celebrating his 80th birthday and also his 50th wedding anniversary. The reporters gathered around him to express congratulations. Then they asked, "What do you attribute this long span of successful living to?" He reflected for a moment and replied, "When I got married my wife and I had an agreement that any time we saw an argument coming on, I would grab my hat and walk four times around the block. You'd be surprised what 50 years of outdoor exercise will do for your health."

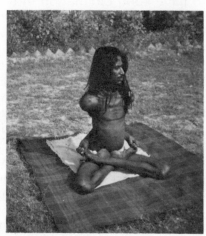

Yoga, India

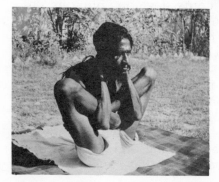

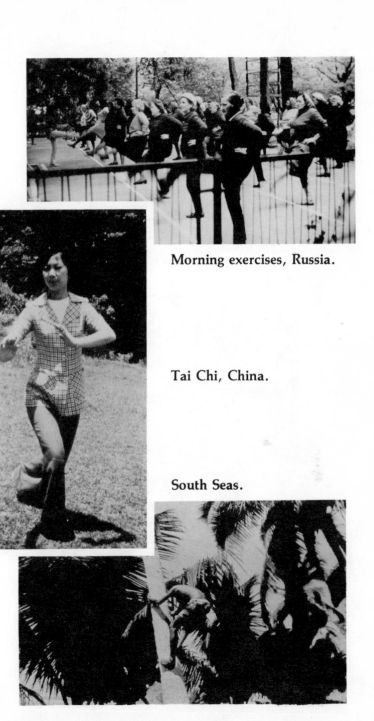

Morning exercises, Russia.

Tai Chi, China.

South Seas.

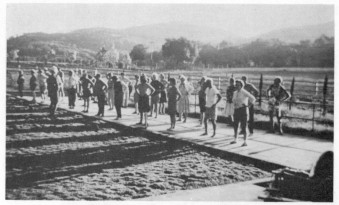

Hidden Valley Health Ranch

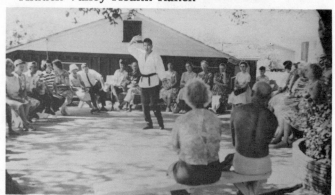

Teaching Tai Chee at Hidden Valley Health Ranch.

Hidden Valley Health Ranch.

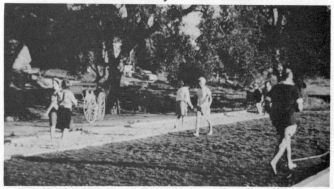

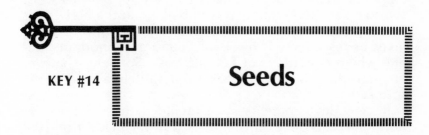

Seeds

I believe SEEDS are the most important food for sustenance. They are Nature's vehicle of perpetuity. In fact, seeds are one of the most LIVING foods known to man—and so are one of the most perfect. Seeds have been found in Tutankaman's tomb, 3,000 years old. Upon planting, these ancient seeds sprang to life!

Even the giant redwoods grow from tiny seeds. All the life-giving elements are there, carefully locked in. Seeds contain nearly every single food element discovered—and doubtless most others ever likely to be. They are of highly potent therapeutic value. The Hunzas claim that the apricot *seed* is partly responsible for their long lives. In the animal kingdom it is said that the seed-eating species, such as the squirrel, are more intelligent than other kinds. Some doctors believe that the high nutritive value of seeds helps the human mentality. So be it, they are 20 times richer in phosphorus than fish, always hailed as a brain food.

The plant gives all it has to the seed, so that even if grown on poor soil seeds are still rich food. But, of course, the better the soil, the better the seed. Highly mineralized, organically treated, unsprayed soil grows the best seeds.

Seeds are the highest protein food in the vegetable kingdom, and contain nearly all the 10 essential amino acids. In many respects they outdo meat. They are rich in the Vitamin B complex for nerves and muscle coordination; Vitamin E for the heart and reproduction—the two elements sadly missing in refined foods of today. Vitamin F for skin and hair health, and the other anti-cholesterol factor, lecithin, are both highly present in seeds. Being low in sodium, those on a salt-free diet can partake of seed foods without fear. Calcium for bones and teeth, magnesium for the bowel and processes of birth, and potassium, the healer, are all present in seeds in goodly amounts. Silicon, the magnetic element for our alertness, is also essential if Vitamin B is to be held in the body. This is found on the outside of seeds. The fluorine in seeds gives us resistance. It has been found an important mineral where conditions of fall-out exist. So from whatever angle we look at them, seeds are definitely a food of the future.

Recent developments have included the discovery of hormone substances in seeds. A powder made from the date pit is being used as a source of male hormone, while citrus seeds contain the female hormone.

Beware of man-produced "seedless" fruits. Hybrids haven't the same potency as their original brothers. When seeds are removed, the gland structure is removed, and we no longer have a "whole" food. The food is degenerated. The more seeds, the greater the food's value. Think of the wild strawberry—full of seeds but infinitely delicious. How often are we let down by the lack of flavor of modern plump, almost seedless berries.

SESAME SEEDS

The sesame seed is among the richest of seeds, with a long history as a valuable item of diet. The Turk's strength and endurance has been credited to the sesame seed, which holds an important place among their foodstuffs. Although soy beans have been boosted as the best source of lecithin and used commercially for its manufacture, all seeds are high in this nerve fat, especially sesame seeds. They are excellent for tired, run-down and sleepless people. Sesame seeds are also rich in calcium and Vitamin E and have an alkaline reaction.

They can be used whole sprinkled over foods, but more of their value is absorbed if they are ground into a meal. The seeds may also be liquefied into a highly nutritious, easily-digested milk. This milk may even be left to sour and then strained to make a vegetable cheese which is less putrifactive than regular cheese.

SESAME MEAL

This is an excellent source of protein, especially as this protein contains all the major amino acids found in meat and in comparable proportions. (See table.)

AMINO ACIDS IN SESAME MEAL AS COMPARED WITH MEAT

Amino acids	Sesame meal (%)	Meat (%)
Lysine	2.8	10.0
Tryptophan	1.8	1.4
Methionine	3.2	3.2
Phenylalanine	8.0	5.0
Leucine	7.5	8.0
Isoleucine	4.8	6.0
Valine	5.1	5.5
Threonine	4.0	5.0

SESAME OIL

A highly digestible, less-acid-forming oil than olive or any other common vegetable oil is cold-pressed, virgin sesame seed oil. Being unheated and unrefined, it is very flavorful and high in its original vitamins. Try it as an excellent skin salve as well as a tasty salad oil.

Sesame oil is not widely known in the United States, but in Central and South America, Asia and Mediterranean countries it is considered a superior edible oil because of its high quality and stability. This stability is due to the powerful anti-oxidants released upon its extraction, especially its high content of a strong anti-oxidant called sesanol.

Average oil percentages range from 47 to 56%, and this is made up of the fatty acids:

Palmitic acid	6—12%
Stearic acid	2— 9%
Oleic acid	32—49%
Linoleic acid	35—52%

comparison of the fatty acid composition percentage of the oil of corn, sesame and safflower.

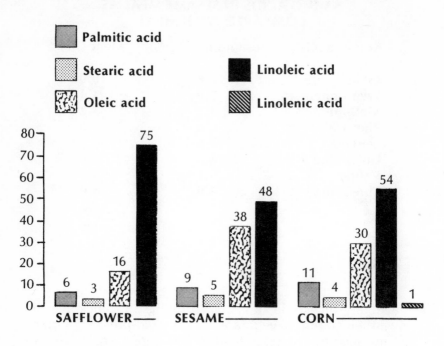

- ▨ Palmitic acid
- ▦ Stearic acid
- ▧ Oleic acid
- ■ Linoleic acid
- ▤ Linolenic acid

SAFFLOWER — 6, 3, 16, 75

SESAME — 9, 5, 38, 48

CORN — 11, 4, 30, 54, 1

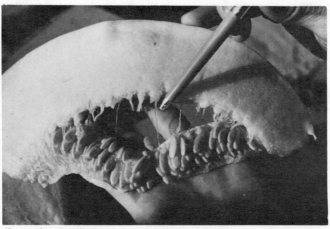

One third of the squash and melon is comprised of seeds. Always use them because they are an excellent source of protein.

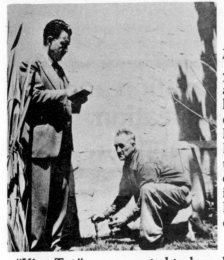

After being apparently "dead" for thousands of years in King Tut's Tomb, ancient peas have come to life in the vitalizing soil of our times. Above left, Jay R. McCullough, curator of the Rosicrucian Egyptian Museum, directs the chief gardener, P. D. Howland, in planting the seeds in Rosicrucian Park. The seeds are direct descendants from original

"King Tut" peas reported to have been taken from the tomb of that Egyptian king by Mr. Howard Carter, who was a member of Lord Carnarvon's expedition in 1922 and 1923. The first planting of the seeds was in England under the sponsorship of Lady Gilbert to whom Howard Carter gave them. The first of these peas were eaten on January 29, 1945, and proved to have a very appetizing flavor.

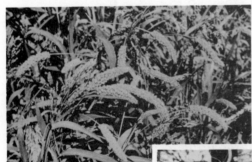

Millet seeds of Hunza. This is one of the best strength builders I found in Central Europe and the Hunza Valley.

Seed in Arabia. This gives them most of their protein for strength and energy.

Relaxation and Recreation
[Strain and Stress]

REST

It was Solomon who said we should work eight hours a day, play eight hours a day, and rest eight hours a day. Of course, to most people, rest means sleep. The elderly people, when the day was finished, didn't have too much of the life we do in the city. We talk about City Lights and the Great White Way, the Broadway of New York, that keeps people going into the wee hours of the morning. Without electric lights they go to bed early.

One of the things I know, from a health standpoint, is that the hours before midnight, in bed and sleeping, mean more towards recuperating your health and keeping you well, than all the hours that you can sleep after midnight. The old saying, "Early to bed, early to rise, keeps a man healthy, wealthy, and wise," still holds true today.

We produce an acid condition in our bodies in the presence of light. Light makes our body active, It makes it move. There is a lot of repairing to be done whenever we live, or just sit, in the light of day. Sunshine makes our body active, but darkness produces a lassitude, a relaxation, a negative influence and our body just folds up. We find that it is supposed to just let go. This is the time of the day for meditation. This is not the time of the day for activity. Action should come in day light. Man is a day animal, he is not a night animal. We produce acid conditions in the daylight and in the night, in darkness, we produce an alkaline condition. The more time we spend sleeping before midnight, the more we alkalize our bodies. Many of us produce acid conditions in our bodies through mental activity and not enough sleep, that all the alkaline broths can never replenish. There is no artificial darkness. The sunshine can penetrate the earth's surface 250 feet.

Sometimes we wonder why with the extra sunlight, the people living in the arctic shouldn't have better bodies or live a longer life. We find that the reflections from the sunlight against water, against the snow can be very harsh on the body. For instance, you can look at the way man has been built. It is only the upper lid that comes down to keep you away from sunshine. The under lid does not keep you away from the reflections of snow and water. That is why we can have sun blindness. This is why, many times, people can take a vacation out on the water and get water blindness from the sun's reflections against the water to the eyes. These people have to develop an extreme amount of pigments in the body to keep away from the reflections of sun and the sunshine itself. This can also draw on the body's resources in order to do this. We don't find any long-lived people in the South Seas who have a lot of sunshine.

On the other hand, we don't want to get to the place to where we believe that sunshine has the *answer* to long life. They may not have all good foods up in the arctic, and they may not have all the best foods in the tropics. We have already told about the top soil in the tropics, and in the arctic they don't have any topsoil at all. They have to depend upon other things. The only thing that they have there in the arctic in the way of topsoil foods is the food they find in the stomach of the walrus when they kill him. These are the only greens they can get. A great book was written one time by Dr. Cabot, "What Man Lives By". He says we live by work, play, rest, and love. Here is a medical doctor to tell us the four things we live by.

Rest is a cure. A tired body cannot get well. A tired body cannot eliminate. A tired body cannot repair or rebuild. It cannot rejuvenate unless it has vital energy to work with. The rested body is the one that gets well. Many times the person who gets sick is the one who has overworked and is trying to conquer his impatience; he learns life's accomplishments are not so all-important after all, or having to get things done to satisfy his ego, or possibly his pocketbook.

In New Zealand they have more of a vacation time, or what they call a holiday time. From Friday night to Monday morning, it's their holiday. Everyone is out in the ocean, in the water, down at the beach, fishing, playing and away from their work. This holiday has given New Zealand something to think about. They have more people there that live a longer life on an average, than any other country in the world. The average person in New Zealand lives to the age of 79. No other country, when you look at the whole population, can say they live to that age.

WORRIED TO DEATH
[Copied from a newspaper item]

Automation worried Horace Moulds to death. Moulds worked in a sugar refinery in a department employing 52 girls. And there was music piped in for everyone to enjoy.

Then one day two huge machines were installed. They did the work of all 52 of the girls and they were all fired. Moulds was left alone in the department. And the music also was eliminated. Now there was only the noise of the machines.

The 53-year-old Moulds began to worry about his job. Before leaving for work the morning of last June 4th he told his wife, May, "I've got to make up my mind soon. I'll either have to learn to live with the machines or get another job."

But he didn't go to work. He went to some railroad tracks near his home in Rolleston, England. Then he waited until a train sped by at 60 mph, and he threw himself to his death under its wheels.

TENSION—RELAXATION

We can stand only so much tension, but most of us are in a state of tension all of the time and think we are getting by with it. When you go to the doctor's office he gives you a tranquilizer for tension. When you are too tense, he has to give you a shot to knock you out. One out of every ten persons in this country is using tranquilizers. 300 billion tranquilizers were sold in this country last year. That is a lot of 'dope'.

Most of us carry tension in our bodies all of the time. We should know how to relax and let go. In order to really relax, you must consciously tense more and then when you can't hold it any longer, relax. Then you will have complete relaxation; then the nerves can recuperate. You cannot recuperate with semi-tension in the body all of the time. We get rid of it by tensing more and then succumbing to complete relaxation. Practice this tension-relaxation regularly; if you relax properly once in a while, the body can recuperate very quickly.

Many people go to bed thinking they can relax, thinking sleep is going to help them. Many times they wake in the morning just as tired as when they went to bed. You can recuperate only when you relax; so to release body tension and let the blood flow freely, relax; let go. In order to do this we must walk with an entirely different attitude toward life. To let go is to "let God"; that is, we stop trying to *make* life happen. Find what a good life is and allow it to flow through. Meet life with a good body, a good mind and a good spirit. Meet any problem that way and it will be taken care of easily.

Nobody wants sickness. Think of all the people who are worried to death. There is absolutely no happiness in bitterness, no happiness in anger or unrest. People stagger through life and through the years throttled by their thoughts. Some of the people who come to see me are filled with fear and worry. They worry about everything and anything. Give them a project, a problem, something to think about and instead they worry about it. They seem to be 'natural worriers'. We must choose a more healthful way to live.

CHANGE YOUR LIFE

It is the weary and the miserable who die prematurely. You must lift up, you must find your true heritage in life. You must find who you are, what your birthright is. You must follow something in your life; you must transform your life. You must go down the right channel. I have said repeatedly we have to choose the better things in life, so we must choose a healthful way to live. When a problem comes to you, recognize it. Get in and take care of it. That is your time to meet it and you can only meet it with your intelligence quotient, with emotional stability.

For one moment let us analyze the word "to manifest". It means "man-I-feast". How many people 'feast' on the negative things in life! Man-I-feast—manifest. Yes, whatever we see, we express. Do not allow things that are going to distract and disturb you to come into your body. Change your life, but change it from within. Know what it is to walk through life having comfort on the inside. Nothing on the outside can ever give you this comfort—it is closer than breathing. There is something on the inside that can illuminate you and give you the life that is necessary to carry you through all of your problems and troubles.

CONSERVATION OF ENERGY

This is the greatest lesson that we must learn We must know what it is to have a quiet mind. To have possession and to keep possession of your world is important. To know what it is to rest, to get release from tension, to get relief from constant overwork, to have a change, to know what it is to be still, these are the things that will conserve your energy.

A tired body cannot eliminate, absorb, digest, plan, love or concentrate properly. A person who can meditate and develop a quiet time for himself will have the secret of getting well and staying well.

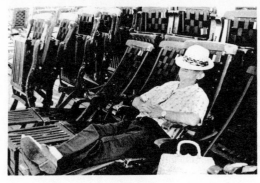

Let go and let recuperation take place.

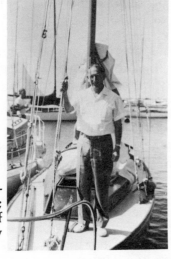

Getting away from it all isn't always just a matter of letting go; sometimes it is involving yourself in activities other than your daily routine.

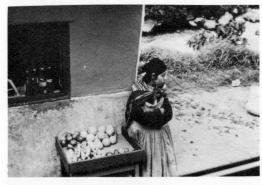

Selling fruit in Central America. When we work without strain our bodies will recuperate properly.

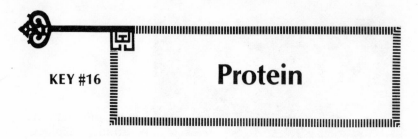

Protein

Protein is the most important food in our food routine. I don't say it is the most important in the diet, but it is the one factor that seems to be lacking in many of the diets throughout the world where we find people living the shortest life.

In India, people live to the average age of 31 or 32 years old, and it is caused by a lack of protein. Eighty percent of their diet is lacking protein.

We went to Helaconia where this photograph was taken of a young doctor and my wife, Marie, with young people coming out of school.

It was in this community where the average person only lived to the age of 30. They lived on raw sugar and corn, and by adding sixty percent of soybean milk powder to their diet, they had cut down the death rate to an unbelievable amount.

The doctors are taking measurements of the children's bones and of people there to show the changes in their bodies. Their life span has now increased so tremendously by just adding a protein to the diet.

All proteins are made up of a small unit, the amino acid. There are more than 20 different amino acids, and the body can synthesize at least 12. This fact was discovered by William Rose, a biochemist at the University of Illinois. Ten amino acids are known as "essential" because they cannot be so manufactured and must be supplied in foods. These ten are: arginine, phenylalanine, valine, lysine, tryptophane, threonine, histidine, leucine, methionine and isoleucine. These must be available for child growth; however, it is probable adults can get along on eight.

Because vegetable proteins lack one or more of the essential amino acids, they are classed as "second-class protein". Animal proteins, on the other hand, have all the essential amino acids (except gelatine, which lacks three), and are called "first-class protein". This classification is rather misleading. With a good variety of vegetable proteins, the vegetarian can obtain all the essential amino acids because any lacking in one food will be made up by others (the total of over 20 amino acids allows for combinations in 2,432,902,008,640,000 different ways!).

Tradition has accumulated a strong prejudice of the inferiority of vegetable proteins. Modern research shows this to be an unsound generalization. Chemically and nutritionally, soybeans, Brazil nuts and peanuts rank with animal protein. It is likely in the near future that others will also class. The very fact that nuts are the only protein of certain tribes in parts of the world, and that millions survive on legumes, poorer vegetable protein, shows that there are gaps in our knowledge. The only essential amino acids found in these in any quantity are isoleucine, threonine and valine. Monkeys and apes (our nearest relatives) live on shoots, berries, tubers, leafy vegetables and nuts; and some of them can shift half a ton. Gorillas are even stronger.

Flesh proteins are acid forming. Practice does not uphold the fact that eating much protein necessarily develops energy and vibrant health. Sometimes the opposite is true.

In 1948 Professor A. Fleisch, President of Swiss Federal Commission for nutrition, stated, "2,160 calories are enough unless a person is a very heavy manual worker (2,400 United Nations minimum daily requirement).

"These conclusions are based on large-scale experiments made with scientific thoroughness on 4,000,000 people in Switzerland. The experiments showed that the amount of calories, proteins and fats formerly considered essential in civilized countries is utterly unnecessary.

"Our conclusion is that a standard figure of 1 gram of protein per kilogram of body weight (0.035 oz. per 2 lbs. 3 ¾ oz.) is correct compared to the more than 100 grams a day advocated before the war, which was not only unnecessary, but harmful."

The body cannot get rid of excess protein but must excrete it by way of the kidneys. Early this century, Professor Russell H. Chittenden of Yale University, carried out thousands of tests on nutrition and proved that the average man eats twice as much protein as he needs. No future experiments have disproved this. Professor Hindhede endorses them. Working with professional men whose occupations were mental rather than physical, he showed that a drastic cut in protein intake improved health, energy and resistance to fatigue. A group of soldiers gained in strength phenomenally. Another experiment was with high-class athletes. He said, "Let us turn our attention for a moment to a group of university athletes, remembering that these men have been training for many months and some for several years prior to the commencement of the trial with a reduced protein intake. In the words of the director of the gymnasium, 'These eight men were in constant practice and in the pink of condition; they were in training when they began their change of diet.'

Some of them have gained marked distinction for their athletic work; one, during the early months of the test, won the collegiate and all-around inter-collegiate championship of America. Compare now the strength tests of these men as taken at the beginning and end of the five-month experiment, during which they reduced their daily intake of protein food more than 50 percent."

STRENGTH TESTS	January	June
W. G. Anderson	4913	5722
W. L. Anderson	6016	9472
Bellis	5993	8168
Callahan	2154	3983
Donahur	4584	5917
Jacobus	4548	5667
Schenker	5728	7135
Stapleton	5351	6833

Carl Voit, a vegetarian, weighing 128 pounds, wrote a book about his experiences in maintaining perfect health on 52.5 grams of protein a day.

Of today's agricultural abundance, Dr. W. A. Albrecht of the University of Missouri says, "We are producing bulk, not quality, and we are paying for it in our own health as well as in the health of plants and animals.

AMINO ACIDS ARE CONSIDERED
THE BEGINNERS OF LIFE

There is a lot of talk these days about our needing more protein in our diet. It is something to think about, especially when people are eating so haphazardly and gambling with their digestion at the corner restaurant, baseball games and drug store counters. We are making a living by straightening out people's dietary habits, teaching them how to live correctly, and setting up new nutritional patterns that they may follow.

One of the most important things to realize is that our bodies must have a new beginning to get out of the predicament most of us are in. Then we must learn a way of maintaining good health. Everyone seems to be dieting these days. Get off a diet. Learn a good healthy way to live. Diets are useful for slenderizing and for the elimination of various toxemias, but let us also reckon with one fact—we must learn how to live correctly after we get off the diet. A basic way of living should include six vegetables, two fruits, at least one starch and at least one protein every day. The average person who really wants to build his body and nervous system should consider adding extra protein value.

Many of the amino acid preparations we have today do not contain all the different amino acids our bodies need. There have been experments which show that glutamic acid is especially good for backward children. Children fed on this amino acid have far surpassed others in tests, showing that it is probably one of the factors missing in the diet, or is needed in larger amounts when such a condition exists. Amino acids have various functions in the body besides being a main component of flesh tissue. Some are specific in action. For instance, one amino acid may assist the gall bladder, another the liver, and still others different organs and expressions of the body. In order, therefore, not to run the risk of missing any essential factor, it is well to get a variety of proteins. Do not depend upon any one protein for all the amino acids. Soy beans probably have most of them—but not all—and to rely on soy beans entirely would lead you to find weakness in your health over a period of time due to this lack.

It has been said that a person weighing 175 pounds would need 85 grams of protein a day, or the equivalent of one half pound or 2 cups. But it is foolish to say that these figures can be followed exactly, as there are no two people alike, either in physical make-up or temperament. Highly-strung persons would no doubt use more than the calm, serene types. Tension, worry and fretting wear one out. The person who has found a tranquil way of living will not have to depend on food to pay back shortages in his body or build up a burnt-out chemistry in organs or tissues. So you cannot treat everybody exactly the same.

Now, if you feel you need something in writing to fol-low, here is a table to help you. Personally, I believe that our protein intake is too high and we would do better to learn a way of living that would allow us to get along with much less protein in our bodies. But, in this day and age of horseracing, tranquilizers and ant-acids, people need immediate help while learning a better way to live.

The most natural way to correct any of your bodily problems is to consider using the following foods because their protein is rich in amino acids. It is well to use two, three or four of them daily, in the amounts suggested, in a glass of tea, pineapple or any other juice. This makes an excellent protein tonic. Vary the drinks from day to day. Sweeten them with a tablespoonful of maple sugar, apple concentrate or grape concentrate.

Lecithin . . . . 1 tbsp

Lecithin . . . . 1 Tbsp
Gelatin (pure beef) . . 1 Tbsp
Wheat Germ Flakes . 1 Tbsp
Wheat Germ Oil . . . . 1 Tbsp
Brewer's Yeast . . . . . . 1 Tbsp
Vegetable Broth
      Powder . . . . 1 Tsp
Egg Yolk 1
Soy Milk Powder . . . . 1 Tbsp
Dried Milk Powder . . 1 Tbsp
Skim Milk Powder . . . 1 Tbsp
Raw Milk . . . . ¾ Glass
Yogurt . . . . 2 Tbsp

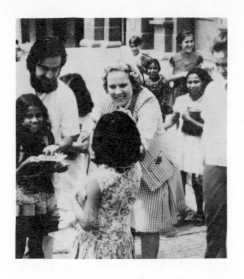

In Helaconia the average life span was age 30. After protein, in the form of soy powder, was added to their diet the life span was increased. The doctor in this picture was most kind in showing us the medical records indicating the increase in the span of life from just the addition of protein in the native eating habits.

From China . . . .

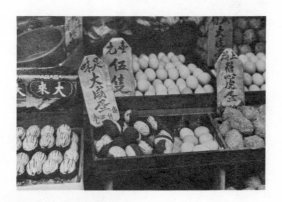

. . . France . . .

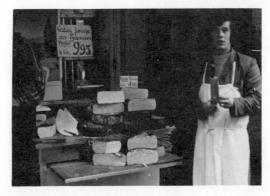

Switzerland,

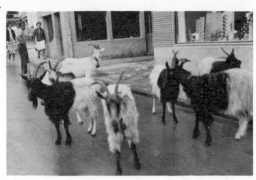

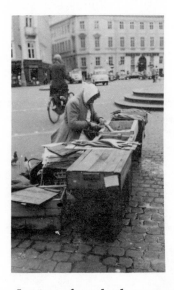

and Denmark, we find protein used in the forms of milk, eggs, fish, cheese is an important part of diet.

It was found that people in India were short up to 80 per cent of the necessary proteins in their diet.

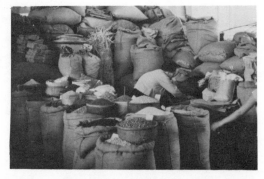

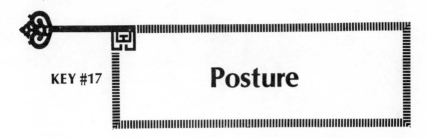

KEY #17

Posture

The National Chiropractic Association sponsors a National Correct Posture Week from May 1st to May 7th. This has been observed each year by the chiropractors throughout the country. This first week in May is a very important one for good health. It was noted by the Chiropractic Research Foundation that thirty-five per cent of all adults have spinal defects likely to lead to organic disease unless corrected.

Standing tall, sitting tall, and walking tall should be our uppermost thought for good posture. Posture habits are formed early in life and these three points should be considered in training and raising our children. The following rules will help in this training.

FIRST: Learn to stand tall, sit tall and walk tall.

SECOND: Follow a few simple daily exercises to preserve strength and tone of the ligaments and muscles which support the spinal column.

THIRD: Learn to relax completely.

It is recognized that good posture is the foundation of good health. We find that in correct posture we allow the different organs of the body to have free movement with one another and no pressure symptoms are produced on one organ more than another. The knees do not become buckled, prolapsus does not set in, shoulders will not droop and the Adam's apple will not be pressed forward to put pressure on the thyroid gland. Our breathing becomes deeper with good posture. Our chest is carried higher. Good posture does away with lower back curve and the consequent curves that develop in the upper

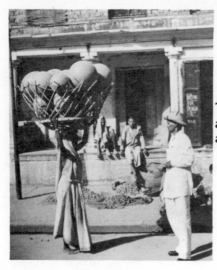

This posture is to be desired, as in India carrying loads on an erect body.

spine. With good posture we walk with our feet straight ahead; the muscles of the legs are strong, the veins and arteries carry the blood more freely and the nerves in our body carry the messages from our brain to the different organs without any inhibitions or stimulation. Digestion and elimination are improved through good posture.

Calcium is essential for the formation of bones, and we find that it is one of the chemical elements we usually lack. Teeth have been straightened and become firm in their sockets, and the gums have changed their appearance just through adequate feeding of calcium. We develop small jaws because we lack certain mineral elements which causes an improper balance of those elements already present. We also lack exercise.

According to the U.S. Department of Agriculture, calcium is essential in poultry diet for the maintenance of the hatchability of the egg. Calcium affects the thickness of the shells and their resistance to breakage. A chicken can draw on her skeleton for enough calcium to make only three or four eggs. A hen that lays 200 eggs per year puts into those eggs many times more calcium than she has in her body, so she must be given the proper calcium replacement. At Petaluma, chickens are fed green kale, which is high in calcium, so that the eggs will have a hard shell. These eggs are sent all over the world so they need a hard shell to resist breakage. They also use coquina shells (calcium carbonate), which are very high in calcium.

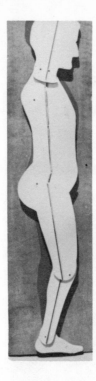
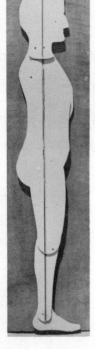

Keeping the body erect, walk like the upright man, with a straight line right down through the center between the ears, shoulders, hips, knees and ankles.

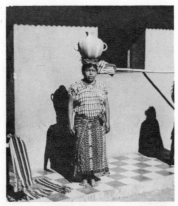

In Central America you see so many of the people carrying pottery on their heads when they are walking. They have beautiful postures. I never met a bent old man.

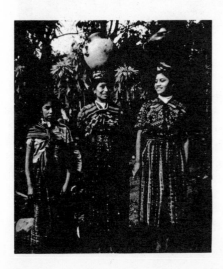

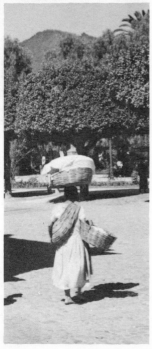

KEY #18

Beauty—in Color, Art, Music

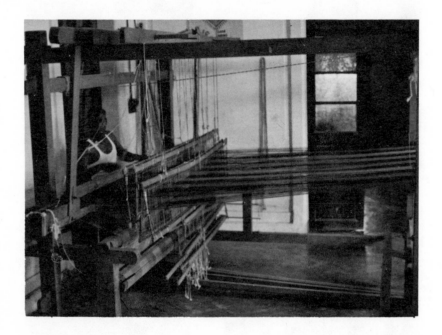

BEAUTY AND COLOR

The older people throughout the world looked for beauty and color. This they wove into their fabrics. The color they used is expressed through their vegetation. They knew, and taught me that it is the yellow vegetables that are laxative. It is the blackberries that produce a constipating effect when a person has diarrhea. They used the various colors of these vegetables for healing. They knew the value of beauty. When you talked to them, they told about their high mountains that go up to reach the blue sky. They were poetic about their surrounding beauty.

MUSIC

Music is very important. Whenever there was a lack of music the people would develop it in some way or another. For instance, when Africans were brought to the Virgin Islands they could not use the African drums. They started making drum music out of oil cans and out of gasoline drums that were left there after the war, and this is where drum music was developed. It is said in France, that wherever there is music there are happy people. People can't live in misery. They have to be happy. Man was created for joy. Music is the universal language everybody understands. When music is played everybody reacts to it. Music has been used to bring harmony among people, and harmony is one thing that is conducive to long life. Where there is chaos, there is destruction of good feeling. Music always brings good feeling along with it.

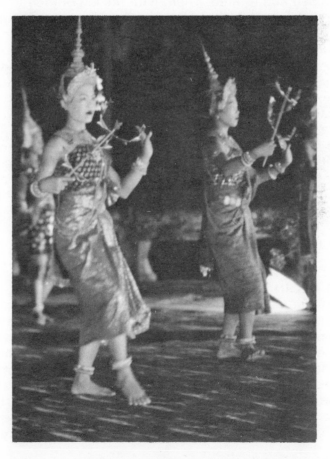

"I AM MUSIC"

by A. C. Inman

Most ancient of the ancient arts; I am eternal. Even before life commenced upon the earth, I was here—in the wind and waves. When the first trees, flowers, and grasses appeared, I was among them; and when man came, I at once became the expression of man's emotions. When men were little better than beasts, I influenced them for their good.

In all ages I have inspired men with hope, kindled their love, given voice to their joy and sorrow, cheered them on to valorous deeds, and soothed them in times of despair. I have played a great part in the drama of life, whose end and purpose is the complete perfection of man's nature. Through my influence human nature has been uplifted, sweetened and refined. Then, with the aid of men, I have become a Fine Art. From Tubaleain to Thomas Edison, a long line of brightest minds have devoted themselves to this perfection of instruments through which men may utilize my powers and enjoy my charms. I have myriads of voices and instruments. I am in the hearts of all men and on their tongues, in all lands and among all peoples; the ignorant and unlettered know me, not less the rich and the learned.

For I speak to all men, in a language all understand. Even the deaf hear me, when they listen to the voice of their soul. I am the food of love. I have given men gentleness and peace, romance and excitement; I have led them on and through heroic deeds. I comfort the lonely and harmonize the discord of mind—I am a necessary luxury to all men. I am Music.

FIND JOY IN COLOR—MUSIC

Color and music contribute to happiness. Wherever there is color, wherever there is music, you will find happy people. Color can put some people into ecstasy; music delights others. When certain music is playing, look around and you will see toes tapping. It does something to the body; we are carried along with it as there is spirit in music. There is spirit in color, too. We find some colors stimulating as we find certain music stimulating; other colors are sedative to the body, even tranquilizing.

We have all witnessed the effect of a band playing a stirring march. Men have come under the influence of martial music and have done amazing things. I had a friend in the English army, Captain Murdo McDonald Baine, who told me that he had the experience of seeing men really, practically dead come alive suddenly and stand up on their feet at the sound of Scotch bagpipes playing their National Anthem. These boys, with their energies miraculously restored, would pick themselves up and start marching to this music! It gave them a surge of spirit that nothing else could have mustered into their depleted bodies.

We find that music can bring tears, joy, laughter. It can affect the whole gamut of man's feelings. Color can do the same. That's why clothes are so important to us. We pick out clothes as much for the color in them as for the becomingness of style. I've had some suits of my own that I liked and others that I just didn't like, yet they were all practically the same style. A brown suit, for instance, I wore only two or three times and then gave away. I didn't feel good in it; I didn't feel at home in that suit of clothes. A lot of people go through life at home in a spectrum of colors, but they don't know it. We have what are called "colorful moods"; we talk about being green with envy, about red-hot mamas. We know people who sing the blues, and we find people who look at the world through rose-colored glasses. Stop and think about it. We all live in color.

GEORGE CUKOR, FAMOUS FILM DIRECTOR, LOOKS AT BEAUTY:

"I think all women can make themselves lovely—by the way they think, their walk, their voice, their behavior. A lot of a woman's beauty and excitement comes from the inside. I think that beauty is built up cell by cell; it is built up from the inside. It's character, it's warmth, it's a way of thinking; it's knowing the world, knowing and understanding people."

Eliza Doolittle, in "My Fair Lady" had a wise insight into beauty: "....the difference between a lady and a flower girl is not how she behaves but how she is treated. I shall always be a flower girl to Professor Higgins because he always treats me as a flower girl and always will, but I know I can be a lady to you (Pickering) because you always treat me as a lady and always will."

You can make anyone more beautiful if you treat them that way.

VIBRATION AND COLOR

Now there is a 'heart beat' in fruits and vegetables. We can go into the vibratory field; many things will show us that nature has set up something in this world of phenomena that we should get acquainted with. It may be hard to believe that music is vibration, or to believe too, that color is vibration. We live in a world of vibration, where so much is related that we can even change color to music and music to color.

You must realize that color has an effect on your body. Nature has planned the green, the yellow and the red fruit for a definite purpose. There is more Vitamin D in the red than in the yellow, but when you want a lot of Vitamin C, go to the yellow fruit. If you want a laxative, go to the yellow foods. All the good laxatives come from these. Castor oil is yellow; so are peaches and apricots. Nature has prepared and planned these things. Wouldn't it be nice if we knew her well enough to take care of ourselves? But we have not made a study of these things. Every home should know what the laxative foods are and how to get them.

We should all have an herb garden. Why, your whole back yard should be scented with these aromatic herbs which have a wonderful value. It is not a matter of just growing a tree—it should be a useful tree. If you have pine trees, you should know that pine needle tea is high in Vitamin C. Using pine needle pillows is conducive to a wonderful sleep. The leaves from many of the trees and plants can be used in your every day living. Why do we have to live a life that is so foreign to the natural one and then try to keep well on drugs, aspirin and tranquilizers, when we could find the answer in Nature?

Now, of course, there are a lot of people who just don't care. But in the very near future, things will be brought forth to show who the people are who care and those who don't. In fact, these people are separating more and more every day. Can't you tell the people who care? The people who will not sell you out; who are sincere with your life? Those who are putting up the packaged foods today are living for what they can get out of you! But they are not really living; they are a dying people. They are dying out. They will have to die out because they are killing themselves by the same mental process that I told you of in the beginning. They are not treating themselves right, not living the life themselves. There is an old saying "If you give a man enough rope, he will hang himself."

I know of people who want to use some fat from the left hind leg of a bear in Siberia to put on certain sores in order to heal them. They go to extremes. Some people are so meticulous about conditions. For instance, I know of doctors who put you in a well of mud, have you face the north and allow you to be there only between 2:20 and 3:00 o'clock every day with certain kinds of people around you. Of all the ideas I have ever heard of! However, on the other hand, each thing does have its effect on us. I know that the mind and prayer have an effect, not only on the body but on fruits and vegetables to such an extent that they won't even grow; or you can double the growth of plant life through the suggestions you put on it. I have pictures just 'out of this world' illustrating how you can handle plant life by blessing it and by having a good thought toward it. Put any plant on a window sill and it will turn itself toward the sunshine. It needs it. But if you put jazz music next to a plant, it will turn away from it. It has no need for that. Plants are very sensitive to the good. They will respond to you, especially if you are the type who is sensitive to natural things and get along with them.

KEY #19

Harmony and Balance

In the light of knowledge there is a time in life when we come to certain realizations. The majority of the things we realize today have come out of necessity. Most people do not walk across the street fast enough until a horn blows or until an automobile just misses them. Many people do not learn anything about themselves or their health until they have lost it and often this is too late.

Knowledge comes to us when we are capable of accepting it and not at any other time because of circumstances and because our insight would not be able to grasp it. I heard a mother say, that after she had raised her children, she then knew how to raise them. Why should she have the knowledge then, when she needed it in the beginning? We should always seek to acquire knowledge, especially in this day of civilization when there are so many things that are not exactly good for our health and well being.

We have to learn discrimination, to pick out the things that are good for us. Above all things, we should know that our bodies are subjected to the laws of nature. The more knowledge we have of these laws the better we are equipped to keep ourselves in good health. We are subjected to the rhythm of our heart beat. It is when our heart does not beat normally that we realize something is wrong, so we must know what it is to be in harmony with the rhythm that nature has set up for us.

We are also subjected to the cycles of the seasons. There are certain foods that we must eat at certain times of the year. We should learn more about the law of cycles and live according to them. Air, food, water, exercise should come in our living habits, but where? Let find out.

Mental happiness and spiritual growth bring power and iov that most of us seek. Let us take time out for self-realization. You are the center from which all these laws emanate. You are the most important person in the world.

THE WHEEL OF LIFE

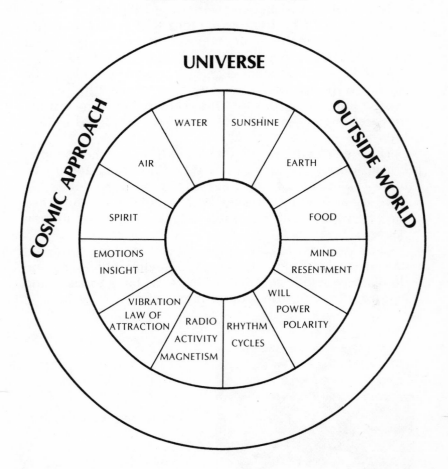

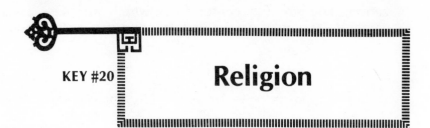

KEY #20

Religion

These long-lived people were very religious; they believed in a divinity. Some didn't look to it as God, but they lived close to nature and believed there was a greater force that held them together and gave them life.

In their religion they had certain structures built within it, that were conducive to long life. Most of those who lived a long life were Moslems. They believed in fasting, moderation, they didn't drink or smoke, they led the clean life.

They led the life where they tried to help other people. Prayer four or five times a day was a necessity and a custom. This is one of the great habits. In our country we have a pause that refreshes with a cola drink, but they have a pause that refreshes: a prayer and meditation pause!

They got close to God during these times and came out of their meditation with a serviceful feeling of helping and doing more good for others as they got back to work and associated with those around them.

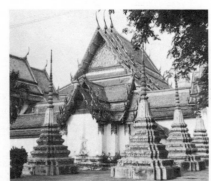

Religion is part of everyone's life.

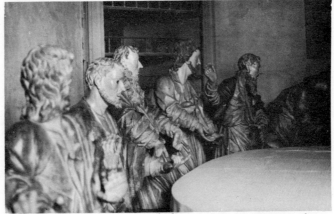

Brazil: When we viewed these statues representing
Christ with His disciples, one in our group pulled a
gun and shot Judas.

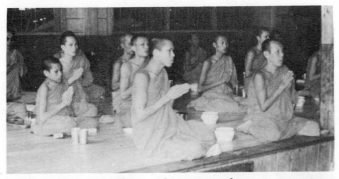

Part of the Buddhist religion is that young men
should give up one year of their lives for spiritual
training.

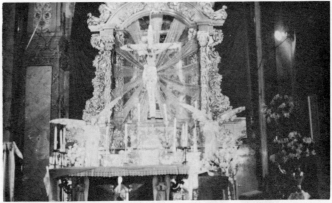

Religion is part of everyone's life.

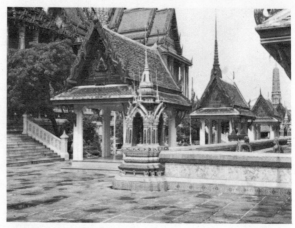

Buddhist temples are beautiful and colorful.

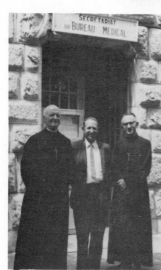

Investigating the faith cure medical records at Lourdes, France.

Prayers sent to heaven on steps of church in Chichicastanango.

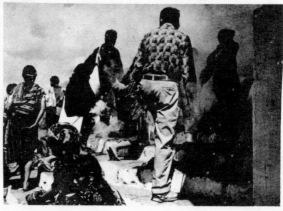

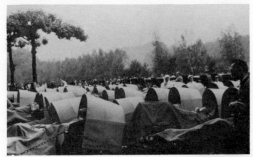

I saw 16,000 people come daily to the Shrine at Lourdes.

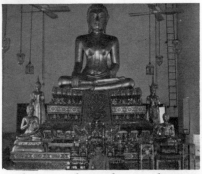

The shrines throughout the world indicate man's need for spiritual rejuvenation.

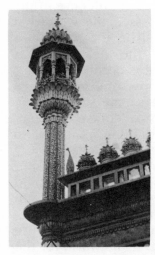

Moslem temple.

Lourdes, France.

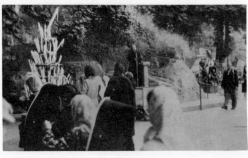

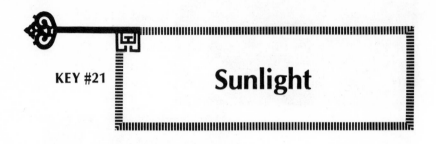

KEY #21

Sunlight

I had a great experience in visiting Leysin in Switzerland. We saw some 4,000 homes with balconies on the outside where people from all over the world came for the sun cure. We should realize that the sun controls the calcium in the body. To have this sun coming through the pure air as found in the Swiss Alps is so necessary to control the calcium. This is where Dr. Rollier, the famous French physician, developed the effective sun cure in the past. The particular thing that impressed me was what he said: "It is easy to get people well in the mountains whenever they are sick because of the clear sun that comes through this rarefied air. There is nothing to interfere with the sun's rays." He had a personal experience that demonstrated to him the value of the sun. At one time his dog has a sore on its back, and of course, his practice was to put a bandage on it; but the dog went over to the door of the house and rubbed off the bandage every time he put it on; and then went out and lay in the sun. The doctor found that in a few days the sun had cleared up this sore. Later, he treated a lady with TB using the sun cure. She got over it completely, and this young lady became his wife and became the inspiration for him to use the sun cure. People come from all over the world for the sun cure, and one of the specific things they use the sun for is the correction of the surgical hip. Most doctors recognize that only surgery can help this problem, but the sun is able to cure it.

We find that Mr. John Ott in the sunlight center in Florida has shown that the smog in the city cuts out 85% of the ultraviolet from sunshine and that the glasses the average person wears cuts out 85% of ultraviolet rays that go into the body. Ultraviolet is necessary to control calcium in the body. Without proper ultraviolet we would get arthritis, hardening of the arteries, etc. Calcium can come out of solution and settle in the joints. It is very necessary to have enough sunshine for good health and for good calcium metabolism. When the sun goes down, or there is no sun, we do not have the balance to keep us in good health or bring us long life.

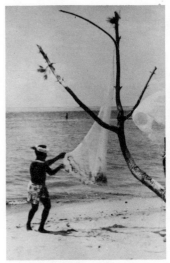 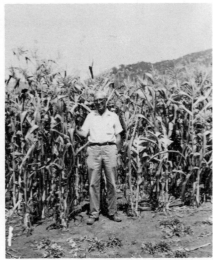

In the South Seas a man works outdoors on his fish nets.

There would be no gardens without the sun.

The sun is brought to each kernel of corn and ripened by way of the tassel.

FOUR CHILDREN KEPT HIDDEN
IN FLAT FOURTEEN YEARS

BOSTON, May 14. (AP)—Children's organizations today pushed an investigation of the case of two Roxbury brothers and two sisters said to have been hidden in a squalid flat for fourteen years because none of them was able either to walk or talk.

Robert C. True, agent for the Massachusetts Society for the Prevention of Cruelty to Children, said the four are offspring of a 73-year-old father and 53-year-old mother, the younger boy is blind as well as dumb, he said, and all are suffering from disease.

The four were patients at Psycopathic Hospital today, pending probable removal to a State institution for specialized training.

Two other daughters, who worked as domestics, supported the family in poverty, since the father was forced to give up his trade as a carpenter, True reported.

A minister's report that neighborhood children saw shadowy figures moving around in darkened rooms of the flat prompted the society's investigation.

When the sun goes down, or there is no sun, we do not have the balance to keep us in good health or bring us long life.

Tranquility

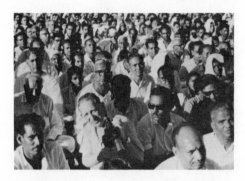

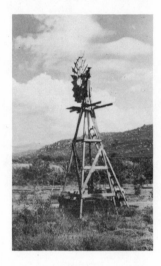

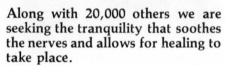
Along with 20,000 others we are seeking the tranquility that soothes the nerves and allows for healing to take place.

I believe that Tranquility is a most necessary Key. We find this quality in the peace and harmony of the mountains; in children at play; in a babbling brook; and in the minds of peaceful men and women.

The very elderly people we met were free of agitation and disturbance. They were very calm, quiet and motionless.

Did you know that one person out of seven in the U.S. is taking a tranquilizer? We know they are taking them for disturbances and for upset conditions. They are anything but composed; they are in a state of alarm. They are aroused and inflamed, highly stimulated and stirring around to such an extent that they have to be stilled. They are agitated and have to be put under control.

However, with the elderly people we found them to be in a state of quiet and with a soothing attitude. Nothing went fast, everything seemed to go in its proper time. They had a still mind and went forward with the idea that things were in good order. They did not overdo their activity. They know that there are rest periods and they follow nature. They go into a period of repose and mental calmness.

They live in an environment that brings about this repose and stillness. When there are fatigue periods that have to be taken care of, we rest in tranquility in a lovely atmosphere that tells us to be still and to know. It tells us to be as the still waters, and this great ability to partake of complete rest and complete tranquility brings about a healing.

There are fatigue periods for all living, breathing beings, and this requires rest and repose. Animals, flowers, plants, trees, machines, even the earth itself has fatigue periods and rest periods, and there are seasons of rest.

Our very hearts have their periods of rest and repose. At night the heart-brain is quiescent and our lungs are almost latent in the extreme activities that are required in the daytime.

Our heart, lungs, heart mechanics, oxidation, brain cells and senses are all in a state of quiescence (motionlessness). Then we cut down perceptibly in our breathing so that many times we wonder, when we see a person sleeping, if he is breathing at all. We don't need as much oxygen at night.

Tranquility fills the mind and soul with stillness; and it throws a placidity over temper and the emotions.

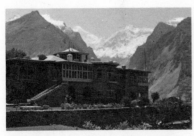

A breeze of tranquility comes over you as you sit on the veranda of the Mir's Palace in Hunzaland. Tranquility talks to you here.

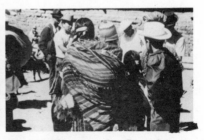

Tranquility can be found in our clothes and in speech. In the markets there is no noise whatsoever.

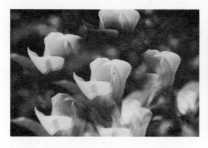

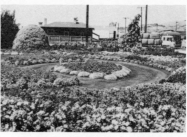

Flowers set a stage where tranquility dances.

Gardens carry a level of tranquility.

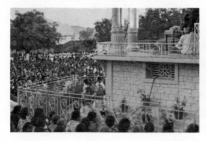

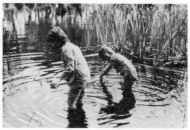

Sai Baba gives out the feeling of a Tranquil Soul and he has millions of followers in India.

Children find tranquility in many places grown up folks have grown out of.

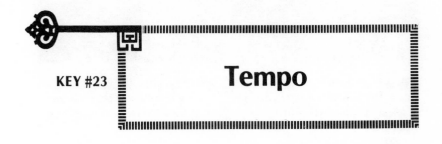

Tempo

I believe we should never have a job that goes faster than our bodies can keep up with it—or, faster than our minds can keep up with it. Many of us are under pressure today. We have to get things out by 5 o'clock. Many a person has finished the day a nervous wreck. Many a person has lived a day that the sleep they got that night could never pay back the energy wasted that day in their job.

We find all the elderly people we know have a philosophy that goes along with their work: you don't have to over-do. I saw one man working who didn't finish his job for the day, and I said, "You only have a few more feet here to finish. Why don't you finish?" He says, "The ground will be there tomorrow." The ground is bigger than he is, and he is going to meet it tomorrow. The philosophy is the great thing as you see it develop here, because we are going into new Keys when we go into the mind. The bodily temple in our daily activities is very important. Never work out the body faster than you can rebuild it.

This has to do with speed and time. We do not enter into the idea that things have to be done by 5 o'clock. We work at the speed of our body and as we can take it.

There is a new disease to be named "gravitosis" and this is very important to consider because I have found that nearly everyone who comes to me is tired, worn out, worn to a frazzle, unable to go, fed up, and can't take anymore. These people are tired physically, mentally and spiritually.

A tired body cannot eliminate; a tired body cannot work; a tired body cannot secrete the proper hormones in the body. This tiredness allows the law of gravity to take over and cause destruction within the body. Prolapsis begins when gravity pulls the lower organs in the abdomen.

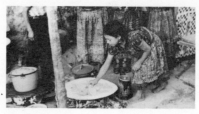

Work at a tempo that will not break down the body faster than you can recuperate.

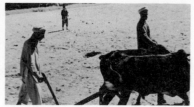

As they plow in the Hunza Valley they keep themselves at an even tempo as they work.

Pressure can build up when one organ is lying on top of another and our tired bodies cannot force blood uphill. It is a tired and fatigued body that is not fit and cannot preserve its life. The stamina is gone and we cannot protect ourselves as an animal can. The tired animal is taken over by the one who is fit and strong, muscularly developed and powerful.

The slanting board is the one thing we have used with our patients for many years to get the blood back into the brain areas. When you study about exercise and taking care of the legs through the Kneipp walk, taking care of the circulation through the lower extremities, then we realize what Dr. Paul Dudley White, Eisenhower's heart physician meant when he said we die from our feet up. It is the legs that bring in the necessary circulation for the brain areas.

We find that the tempo that these elderly people lived at never allowed them to overwork or to do more than what the body could recuperate from with a good night's rest or a good night's sleep.

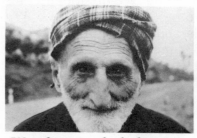

We photographed this 90-year-old man walking into town while visiting Turkey.

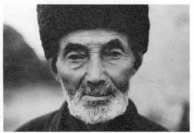

This 100-year-old man in Russia works in the fields with equipment that does not overtax the mind or the body.

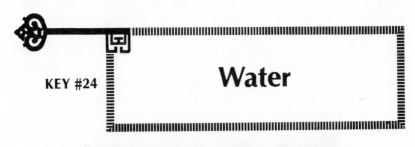

KEY #24

Water

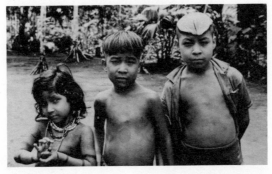

Water can feed or destroy us, leeching the soil and carrying away chemicals necessary for a balanced body. Yet the largest part of our body is made up of water, and the purity of this water is necessary for long life. To illustrate, these children, living in the Amazon, had pigeon chests and curvature of the spine, from lack of a proper chemical balance in the body.

We found the glacier water of Hunza was heavily laden with silt, and was muddy and gray looking; but in the Hunza valley, the Mir himself and everyone there drank this pure water. It was hard to drink because it was so muddy looking, but I do believe, nevertheless, it had mineral elements the body could use.

Wherever these elderly people lived, you find that they never had distilled water. They always drank pure, mineralized mountain water from the glacier peaks and from underground streams. I am not against distilled water, but I feel that they did have a pure, unpolluted natural water as it came from the mountains. The rain water is very important. In some places they even save the rain water to use as pure drinking water.

Most of the people who lived a long life depended a certain amount on rain for their subsistence, especially in their gardens. We have found through experiments that vegetation grows better with rain than with any other type of irrigation. We have all types of water coming through ditches, furrows, and from overhead. There have been many experiments along this line, but it has been found that vegetables and fruits grow much better in aerated rain than by any artificial way of watering vegetation. A good reason why people have better vegetation than we do is because they live in a country where they do not have droughts. They have a good rainfall to take care of their crops.

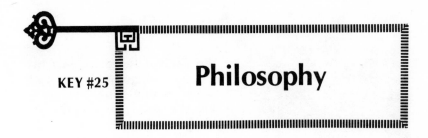

KEY #25

Philosophy

Much has been said about philosophy in the past. Many consider that the mind is Lord of all and that true philosophy is true religion and true science. It is difficult for some to realize how real philosophy can be in living a good life, a long life and a healthy one.

We have looked to the great minds of Lao-Tse, Buddha, Zoroaster, Jesus, the Christ, and others for our philosophy.

Pythagoras, the great moral reformer, who even named himself after the word Philosophos, estimated that there was a study of personal purity and he gave some of the rules in life.

We are convinced that incorrect thinking produces disturbances in the body. There is so much talk about psychosomatic illness today where wrong mental attitudes can cause physical disturbances.

When the physical environment and inheritance comes to us in a balanced, natural manner we have the least need for a philosophy; but when we have obstacles, problems and disturbances we turn to logical thinking and work towards a state of harmony.

I am sure that a good philosophy helps to keep us in a good state of mind.

It was Socrates who gave us the definition of philosophy when he said that philosophy begins when a man picks a carrot out of the garden, eats it and finds that it produces indigestion.

Socrates also said "No man willingly does harm to himself and no man would do bad acts if he could foresee the consequences."

225

It was Plato who long ago prophesied that if a perfect man appeared the world would crucify him. He was right.

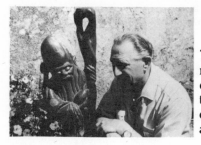

The God of longevity in Chinese mythology holds the staff of life in one hand [representing the good we can do for others], and in the other holds a peach [symbolizing youth].

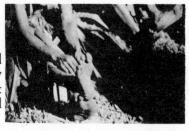

A Fiji Island fire walker. Mind over matter has been used by primitives when they do not have enough of the physical necessities.

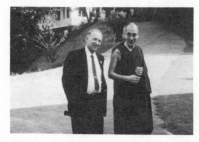

Dalai Lama of Tibet said that our life is limited or extended according to our past lives.

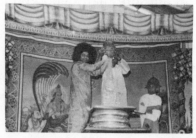

Millions follow Sai Baba for his teachings and philosophy. We need something on which to put our faith while we are searching.

Nervous System

The nervous system has to be taken care of properly. We must recognize that when the cerebellar force breaks down then we develop pain in the nervous system. One way to take care of the nervous system is by feeding it properly, and there are many foods that can take care of the nerves; but the overuse of the cerebellum can break down the nerves.

Pepper, spices, hot and cold foods help to destroy the nerve ends and the nerves themselves. Uric acid will lead to nerve pains and sunstroke, because it affects the nervous substance, especially in the axis cylinder cells of the spinal cord. Extremely cold weather, inflammatory changes in the body, diseases, fevers, a lack of vitality, lack of sexuality and depleted sexual glands, all break down the nervous system. Early decay comes on. When there is mental and bodily weariness, headaches, noises in the ears, dizziness, sleeplessness, exhaustion, general debility, hysteria, disturbances of the sexual system, these all tend to break down the nerves and have to be taken care of properly.

We find that there are many things that are favorable in helping the nerves: altitudes that are not too high or too low are conducive to the rebuilding of the nervous system and to keeping it in good order. Nerve stretching and a change of environment may be necessary. We find that these elderly people always lived in a good environment. They had fresh air, rest, recreation, protection for the body, a good skin activity (working enough each day to carry off the toxic wastes); they used their feet and the vital parts of their bodies were protected from the elements. Regular hours are very important for the nervous system to keep it in good working condition. Lots of iron and oxygen are necessary to keep up the nervous system in good order. Damp, cold working weather is not good for the nervous system.

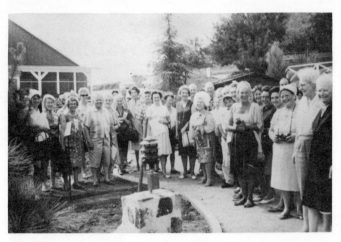

We unburdened our nervous systems by having a burial ceremony for our problems, disturbances, resentments and everyone felt lighter!

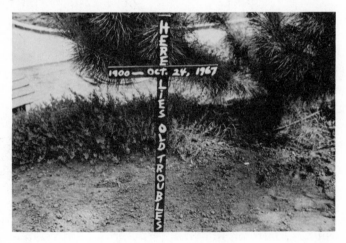

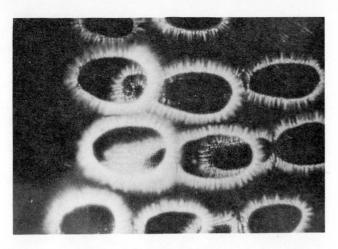

When the nervous system is relieved of problems the free flow of energy is demonstrated by the emanations from the body in this Kirlian photograph. These were photographed at three different times, 1. When I was thinking ordinary thoughts 2. When I was mentally serving people 3. The extreme emanations are when I was in meditation and prayer.

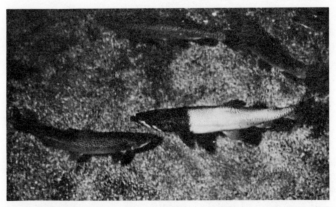

I witnessed one of nature's greatest wonders at Taniwha Springs, Rotorua, New Zealand. The fish shown here were between 25 and 30 inches long, one-half green and the other half brown. When they feed these fish, each is very eager to get his share and fights desperately for his food. I saw the large one, whose name was Harvey, go through a complete change of color. His entire body became brown when he was fighting for his food, but after he had eaten it, his body returned to its natural colors—half brown and half green.

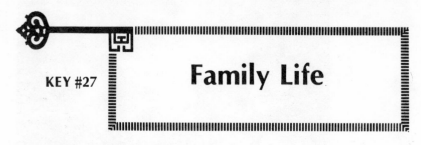

Family Life

It is well we get along with our friends, our family, our neighbors. If we cannot get along with people, we cannot be well. People can cause plenty of troubles. We are afraid of stepping on people's feelings. We don't have to be afraid of stepping on people's feelings if we are developed properly. Everybody is different. You find in all of these elderly people that most of them were the counselors in their towns and were looked up to for what they knew because they had lived long enough to be wise. Their experiences were accepted.

One of the things that allowed them to get along well with others is that they were heavy calcium types. Heavy calcium types are not fast thinkers; they are slow thinkers. They think things over. I feel if we could think things over with one another we wouldn't fly off the handle and our tempers wouldn't rise; we would exercise restraint and think about things, and by the time we counted ten, (which most calcium people do before they think and talk) we probably wouldn't have problems with one another any more.

DESCENDANTS

Most of the elderly people enjoy their descendants and have plenty of them. Their life of reproduction is something they revere and look to. The last man I met at 153 had his last child when he was 120. The man who was 167 had something like 230 descendants: children, grandchildren, great grandchildren and great great grandchildren.

It is a lovely thing to hear these elderly people say, that it is wonderful to live long enough to enjoy your descendants. What grandmother or grandfather doesn't like his children's children?

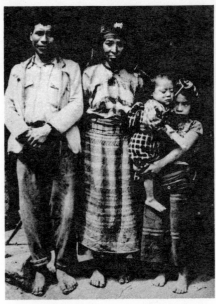

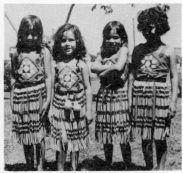

Getting along with one another, as shown by these
Maori children, is really
wonderful.

This shows some people who live
a short life in Central America
where the environment is detrimental to maintaining a good,
healthy body. They lack calcium
and minerals for their bodily
needs. This is demonstrated by
rickets, curvature of the spine,
pronated ankles and pigeon
chests.

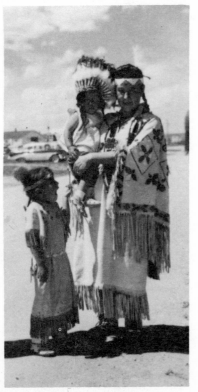

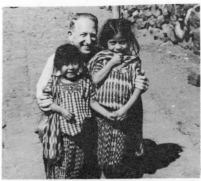

We would like to retain the
youth of a child all our lives, as
evidenced by Central American
children.

American Indian.

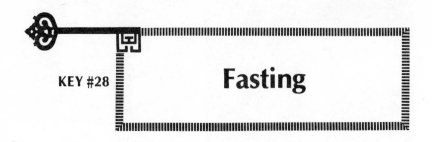

Fasting

The elderly people not only believed in eating, but they believed in fasting. Usually one day a week was set aside to abstain from eating. Once a year they would go to various gatherings and religious festivities and would fast from 10 to 30 days. We have found through experiments with rats that those rats who were fasted and ate only small amounts of food lived twice as long as those who were given all they wanted to eat.

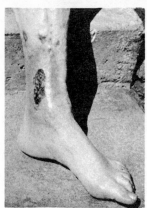

Before fasting

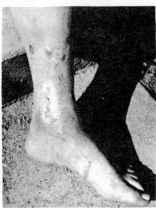

After 10 days of fasting

Fasting has been used for many years by doctors to overcome many kinds of ailments. John Tilden, M.D. of Denver, and Dr. Weger, also an M.D., were advocates of this form of treatment. I studied with Dr. Weger and learned the method of fasting to correct diseases. We are including a few before and after photos of some cases I treated:

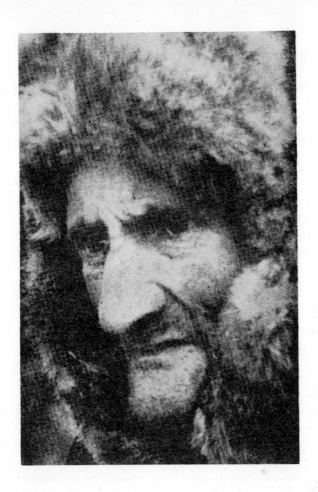

There is a difference between fasting and starving to death. Fasting can prolong life. Many people starve with a full stomach for the minerals they need. A great example is in this photograph.

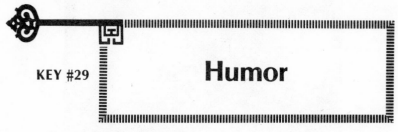

Humor

I tell people to go the lighthearted way, the laughing way, the cheerful way; and we find in so doing that we can give relief to the serious mind, the critical and analytical mind that we constantly use when we are trying to be a success in life.

Humor is very important. Whenever I went to see these elderly people I found them ready for a joke, ready to go the lighthearted way and then return again to the serious way of living.

One of the pastimes for the person who is overworked is to go for amusement to see a show. It is a wonderful and enjoyable experience to see a good comedian. Jokes can be clever and they can be foolish, as people have different ideas about wit and humor. Some people don't want to listen to jokes and think they are foolish, incredible, awkward or unthinkable; but through this faculty we are able to release constant tension. When we use a mental faculty constantly we can wear it out faster than we should. This is especially true if we hang in there a longer time than we should allow any muscle or faculty to work. We have to give every faculty a chance to recuperate.

While in Turkey we found people gathering around in little street scenes visiting each other, drinking tea and having a nice social time. Humor is part of society. I have been to many places throughout the world and everybody knows how to laugh; everybody appreciates a letting-go of the daily routine in this manner.

So long as we can smile and joke we are masters of any situation, even in court.

This reminds us of an actual scene in a courthouse— that of a stern lawyer and an accused malefactor:

LAWYER: "What is you name?"

ACCUSED: "Well, sir, when I was born we were twins, and it being twenty below zero the day we were to be baptized, one of us froze to death, and I cannot just now remember whether it was I or my brother."

LAWYER: (angrily) "Stand down, sir!"

ACCUSED: "I cannot do it; I can either stand up or lie down, but not stand down."

LAWYER: (to Court) "Your Honor, will you kindly make this man answer the questions put to him?"

COURT: (to Accused) "You must answer the questions rightly."

ACCUSED: (to Court) "Very well, your Honor, let him fire away."

LAWYER: "What was your father?"

ACCUSED: "He was humpbacked."

LAWYER: "Well, could he live of that?"

ACCUSED: "He did not die of it."

LAWYER: (angry and roaring) "Are you married?"

ACCUSED: "Certainly!"

LAWYER: (in disgust) "Who are you married to?"

ACCUSED: "To a woman, of course."

LAWYER: (in temper) "Who in high heavens is not married to a woman?"

ACCUSED: "Why, my dear sir, I have a sister that is married to a man."

LAWYER: (confused) "Are you related to this man (a Mr. Smith)?

ACCUSED: "No, sir, he is a Presbyterian and does not have one drop of Quaker blood in him."

LAWYER: (to Court, with tears in his eyes) "Your Honor, I give up."

We have heard many times that "a merry heart doeth good like medicine". How many times have we heart our friends say, "Be of good cheer!" I am sure that the person with the light heart is one who has the best digestion. It is always the serious one, the worrier, and the person who is constantly irritated who develops stomach trouble first.

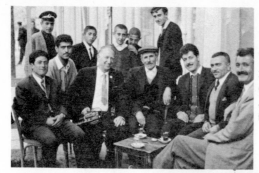

Tea drinking in Turkey is a ceremony that goes on many times a day and is a time for getting together and humor.

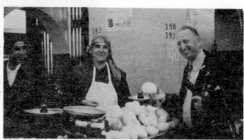

A market in Armenia. It is to work with joy, happiness and a light heart that makes life fuller.

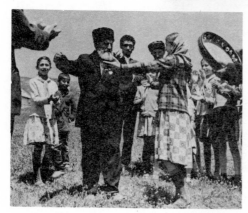

Shirali Mislimov celebrates his 165th birthday with a cheerful note.

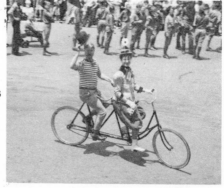

"Smile Awhile—You Kiss Me Sad Adieu."

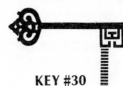

Finances

These elderly people whom I visited all over the world had no finances to worry about. They had no money. They traded. They lived in communities. and whatever one person had too much of, someone else was short of. They were able to barter. It was a lovely way of getting acquainted, to see what your talent was worth, to see the value of a man, to see what his name was worth. What did he put into growing an herb tea, or alfalfa, or corn, as compared to cabbage? How much was the cabbage worth compared to a bushel of corn?

It got to the place that they developed finances comparable to the talent used in growing foods. It wasn't measured dollar by dollar; it was measured talent for talent.

Finances have caused a lot of trouble. I heard years ago if you lose all your money, you've lost a lot; if you lose your health, you've lost still more; but if you lose your peace of mind, you've lost everything.

I don't care how much money you have, how do you control it? A man in Pennsylvania won $125,000.00 in the sweepstakes last year. When he received the news he had only four cents in his pocket. Imagine going from four cents to $125,000.00! What was he going to do? Immediately he started to think of all he could do with this money. For many years he had wanted to own a hotel, so he decided to buy one. Of course, the government got $60,000.00, so he had only $65,000.00 left, but he bought the hotel. One year later he lost the hotel because he didn't know how to handle it. He was so disillusioned, so discouraged, he blew his brains out with a shot-gun. Do you suppose that was worth $125,000.00? Think it over.

I've gone through many of the records of people who have won the sweepstakes. One man became merry, called all of his friends in every night and one year later, he died of alcoholism—all of his money gone. Another man also drank himself to death and died of alcoholism. Each one of these men was made miserable by the money he had won. They didn't know how to handle it.

I think, we have in life what we earn...physically, financially, and mentally. It is a crime to have things in life and not know how to handle them. Let us earn our way. I speak of finances as only one of the many things.

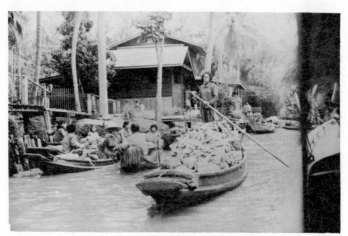

River merchants in Thailand.

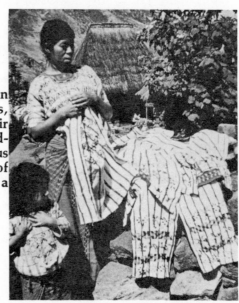

While we are involved in complex banking systems, these people trade their goods and services according to their needs and thus avoid the pressures of finance. I have never met a rich old man.

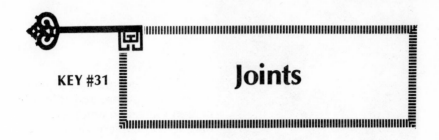

KEY #31

Joints

Sodium is found in nearly all bodies of water and in almost all soils. It is abundant in all plants and plant crops that grow near salty water. One gallon of sea water contains about four ounces of common salt, and this salt is rich in sodium. The sodium salts in plant foods are in an organic form, while those chemically prepared are inorganic. For this reason the sodium compounds obtained from plant foods are better for the body than those artificially prepared.

The principle sodium-containing foods are: celery, spinach, sprouts, strawberries, peas, carrots, okra (very high in sodium), asparagus, figs, Roquefort cheese, goat's cheese, goat milk, goat's whey (this is the highest source of sodium), fish, oysters, clams, lobsters, fresh milk, egg yolk, lentils.

Sodium is present in almost all animal fluids. It is found in the tissues of the human body to the extent of about three ounces. Sodium is the champion acid neutralizer. Because of their alkalinity, sodium salts assist the lymph and the blood, giving these fluids their alkaline characteristics. It plays an important part in the formation of the digestive juices—saliva, bile and pancreatic juices.

Sodium bicarbonate, as found in food, has a beneficial effect on the tissues of the throat, of the naso-pharynx, and on other tissues of a similar nature. Its solvent action helps to remove catarrhal pus, bronchial phlegm, and thick secretions.

Sodium food, in the form of sodium phosphate has a curative effect on gastric and intestinal ailments when there is acidity.

Food, in the form of sodium sulphate, has a curative effect on biliousness, dropsy, scarlet fever, skin diseases,

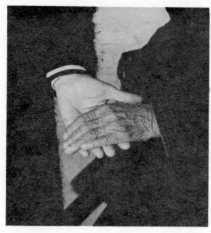

The elderly people had a good balance of sodium and calcium in their diets, and among all the long-lived people I visited during my travels, I never met any who had hardened joints.

enlargement of the liver, vomiting, jaundice and many other conditions.

In warm, sultry weather, sodium salts are used up in great quantities. They are also washed out of the system by water drinking. Heavy physical work calls for more sodium food in the diet.

The functions of the patient suffering from sodium excess, are periodic, as are his diseases. He has thirsty spells, then he may not get thirsty for weeks. At one time his appetite flies, then his hunger is ravenous. His health may be perfect for years, then without any seeming reason, he has a spell of diabetes, indigestion, dysentery, gastrointestinal catarrh, or gout. A girl with sodium excess also goes to extremes. If she dislikes men, or marriage, she becomes a nun. As a reformer, she is a persecutor. When she likes men, she is sometimes an adventuress.

In hot, dry climates, the sodium salts and other alkaline salts are precipitated excessively, resulting in sodium hunger. Sodium hunger produces marked mental characteristics. Such people become depressed, irritable, gloomy and quarrelsome; for absolute sodium starvation leads to erratic mental states. Concentration is poor, memory and recollection defective. Lack of sodium salts produces many striking mental symptoms, such as anxiety, apprehension, gloom, restlessness, a pecular unexplainable longing for something.

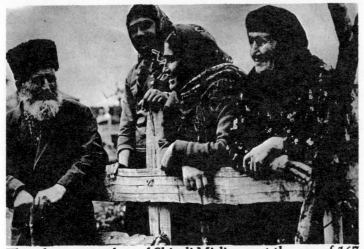

This photo was taken of Shirali Mislimov at the age of 167 with his wife, daughter and granddaughter.

The photo below is of Shirin Gasanov taking home timber for his stove. Both of these men led active lives and kept their joints limber, youthful and pliable through exercises and a good amount of **sodium in their diet.**

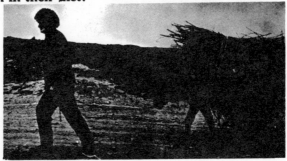

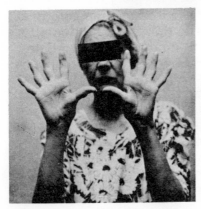

This photo demonstrates what happens when we do not have a proper sodium balance in our bodies.

Schooling

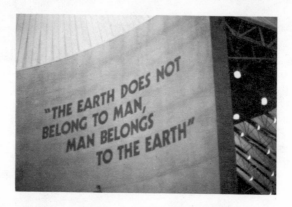

"THE EARTH DOES NOT BELONG TO MAN, MAN BELONGS TO THE EARTH"

I never met an old man who went to school. We find the schooling we have today can make it very difficult for us to live a long life. Many of us have to unlearn knowledge. A trained mind can be dangerous if is hasn't been trained in the art of holding humanity together; if it doesn't have God's principles along with it; if it doesn't have a religious background to be sure you are not skinning the other fellow before he skins you. Man's mind can be dangerous if he doesn't realize that some of the things we are doing to our food, which we call civilized, modern, or up-to-date, can actually destroy mankind—how we are keeping up with the Joneses, or how we are trying to outwit the other person. This is what schools teach. They are not always conducive to giving the other fellow a fair deal. When we deal with the foods today and the many inventions that man has developed, we have to be very careful. I am convinced that man's inventions have come to kill him; and this is because he hasn't developed all the arts of right living, physically, mentally, and spiritually.

A good many things we learned in school, we have had to unlearn. I am of the opinion that there should be a school of the humanities. I personally believe that no school should ever start the day without devoting the first part to considering the rules of life by which we should live.

In our own kitchen we have certain ways of doing things and we have taught people how to take care of themselves through the proper foods, exercise, cultivating a garden, etc., and it is only through these teachings that I see people finding a better pathway to pursue. I feel that the healing art today should be in an educational department.

The average person who has health problems sees a doctor. The doctor is usually too busy today to teach people how to live properly, yet he makes a living on their living.

Isn't it deplorable that doctors should make a living on sick, ignorant people who are eating anything they wish, living the kind of life which brings on disease. Every doctor knows there are occupational hazards, as well as food hazards and hazards in the very air we breathe, but how many inform their patients how to deal with these problems. We must deal with these problems as well as the pollution in our streams.

Our schools need to teach us ways of getting back to nature. We should learn especially how to get along with each other. We should acquire a good philosophy and we should be aware that it is possible to overwork. We should know that we must work and we must earn our way in life.

Above all, we must know there is a right path to take in life. Our soul is crying out for us to get on the path where we may do the right thing for ourselves, physically, mentally and spiritually.

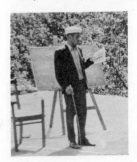

Man must change his concept in schools as to where we belong in nature and what we should learn of the humanities. All the old men I met never went to school.

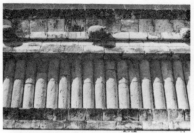

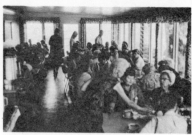

A temple to the turtles where natural living was taught by the Aztecs and the Mayans.

People need to learn how to live so they select good foods at the table of the Hidden Valley Health Ranch.

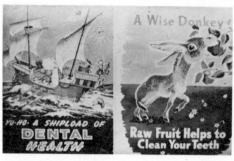

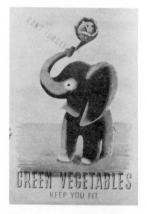

In New Zealand the dentists advertise good health for the good of the teeth.

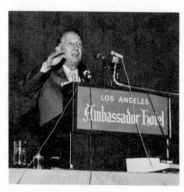

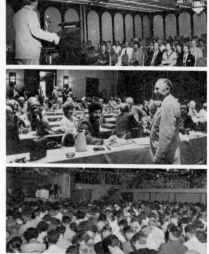

Dr. Jensen has been teaching people the laws of Nature, and how to keep all of humanity together in good health and long life, for nearly 50 years.

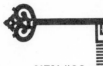

KEY #33

Herbs

These old people drank teas. Not the kind we get in the commercial markets, but they drank the herb teas. They gathered herbs, they dried them, they used them all year round. They used all kinds of herbs.

These herbs afforded them a way of drinking socially. They had as many as 10-12 cups of tea a day and they used them for gatherings and to bring people together. Since these were herb teas, I'm sure they did them a lot of good.

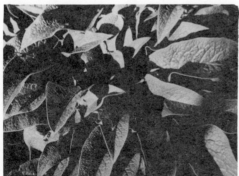

Comfrey is used by the longest-lived people I met.

Natural herbs are used for healing in Hunza.

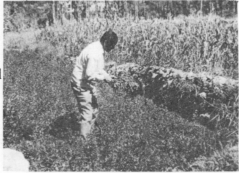

Care of Vital Organs

Vital organs are taken care of beautifully by these elderly people by the way they live, where they live, how they work, etc. We never found anyone who had any trouble with bowels. They have never taken laxatives. They had no inhibitions that produce bowel troubles. The acreage they have around them is their bathroom. They don't have to wait, they don't have to hold it. They don't have to put things off. You find that to go to the lavatory in nature's bathroom is a natural thing for them. I have one lady working for 5 or 6 attorneys who won't go to the bathroom in the daytime because she doesn't want the attorneys to see he take the time off to go. These elderly people don't have these inhibitions. The altitude takes care of their skin. They don't have a dry skin. The humidity is just right in these altitudes. They work hard enough to produce a sweat, to get perspiration going to carry off

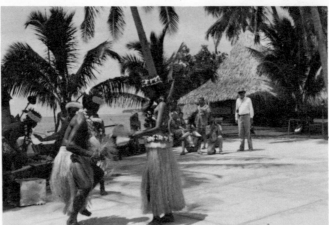

The activity of the day, work or recreation, should help keep up the tone and activity of our abdominal organs. The Tahitian dance certainly does that!

the toxic wastes in their body. They drink the lovely vegetables and fruits they have. I say drink them, because they are so high in water. I believe that the balance of foods they have has exactly, or close to, the amount of water we have in our own bodies. They don't have any concentrated foods like spam, ham, and fried potatoes. All natural foods have enough water to balance the natural water system in our body. They don't have kidney and urinary problems like we do. They don't have any concentrated uric acid problems like we do. When they have fruits and vegetables they are having the same amount of water going into their body as their body is made up of. This is very important.

HEART

The heart is one of the most vital organs with which they have to deal. The heart is never overworked in this altitude or in the work they do. The tempo of their work never overdoes the heart. The exercises of the heart are never too much. They don't abuse this great, vital organ. Also, the lung structure is a vital organ. They live at an altitude where they have to take deep breaths. In a low altitude you don't take a deep breath. The higher you go, the deeper you breathe. They live close to the earth and close to natural foods, they don't live on a lot of the catarrhal-forming foods. Their foods are well-balanced with fruits, vegetables, starches and proteins. However, they don't know that.

As we live in the city we are living on too much bread for breakfast, hot cakes, sandwiches for lunch, then potatoes and bread again for our evening meal. This means too many starches for our evening meal. These could be catarrhal-forming. We also have too many proteins for the day. We have ham and eggs for breakfast or bacon. Or cheese, peanut butter and egg sandwiches for lunch. At night we have to have a steak or a protein meal again. We are having too much of the starches and proteins. I feel that the elderly people balance their diet well because they have so much of the fruits and vegetables with their starches and proteins. This keeps the water circulating well in the body. Water is so important. Most of us dry up when we grow old. Our skin becomes wrinkled and dried. You don't find this in these elderly people. This man of 153 had less wrinkles than anyone I've seen at the age of 60 in this country. I believe it is because they regulate their metabolism by the amount of fruits and vegetables they take inside their body. They take care of the vital organs in the body and this is important to the rest of the body. The shoulder joint depends upon your digestion. The joints in the knees are dependent upon the elimination of the bowels. Every tissue in your body is dependent upon the vital organs.

Chapter 8

Certain Religious Groups

We have become acquainted with certain groups, and I can say that through their religion and spiritual ideas, the basic understanding of life which they teach and which are embodied in their religious concepts, if put into practice, would bring them long life and good health. In fact, we find that in these groups are some of the longest-lived people.

We are going to discuss the Mormons, Seventh Day Adventists and Doukhobors at greater length, but there are other groups I would like to mention that also practice the spiritual precepts and physical ideals to keep them well, healthy and strong. They are the Quakers, the Mennonites and the Amish in Pennsylvania. There are many long-lived people in these groups. You will find much of the substance of our Keys is practiced among these people who are living a simple life and follow many of the principles outlined in this book.

MORMONS

The first group I would like to mention are the Mormons. They have a definite philosophy and definite ideas on how to live physically as well as mentally and spiritually. These precepts give them the best of health; in fact, insurance companies will insure a group of Mormons because they are found to be more temperate, and they are a people who do not drink and do not smoke.

They followed a man by the name of Brigham Young, who I am sure had a lot of calcium in his bones. He was a spiritual man but also had the fortitude and physicality to lead. Brigham Young was a pioneer of the movement who led these people westward. Of course, of those who joined him, many were the mental type; but I am sure that it took much *physical endurance* to carry through and bring those wagons to the west.

These people suffered through many hardships; yet they were able to come through this difficult and trying period. What happened in the Donner Pass and the hardships they endured were almost unbelievable. It takes a calcium body, good health, determination and other strong inherent qualities to succeed in the face of such obstacles.

When Brigham Young came over the pass and looked at the valley, known today as the Salt Lake Valley, he said, "This is the place." I don't know whether it was an inspiration or not, but these people followed him and settled there; and it was the calcium in their bodies that certainly needed the sodium, which was so abundant in that area, to keep their joints limber, pliable and active. It was the one element that was necessary to keep the calcium in solution, in order to keep them young and in good health.

Looking at this valley, we know that it contains one of the most abundant deposits of salt, which has a high sodium content. Everyone has heard about the celery that grows in the Salt Lake Valley. There is no better celery to be found anywhere, and there is no food higher in sodium than this celery. In fact, all foods grown there in the valley are high in sodium. This is where the calcium man should be settling. So when Brigham Young said, "This is the place," it truly was one of the finest places for those pioneers to settle. I might mention that I have examined, diagnosed and analyzed thousands of Mormon people; and they have the finest constitutions, the best recuperative powers, and bodies that can really be well and in good health. I feel that a good deal of this is due to the fact that their religion takes in working with the earth and soil and working with physical things as well as the spiritual and mental. With this type of philosophy, they would particularly attract people who are inclined toward farming, people who want to settle on the land, people with the type of body that has the fortitude necessary to give to the next generation a good physical constitution. I am sure you will find that some of the very elderly in this country will be found in the Mormon settlements and in the Mormon religion.

SEVENTH DAY ADVENTISTS

Another group of people we will hear about more in the future regarding those who live a good healthy life and a long life, are the Seventh Day Adventists. Ellen G. White, the founder of this religious sect, has given much good advice in advocating staying close to the soil, living with the herbs of the field, preventing illness by being people of the farm, leading an outdoor life and taking care of themselves hygienically. These are Keys that can be used along with the spiritual qualities, Keys to balance people in their everyday lives. There are those within the Seventh Day Adventist movement who have left other religions and philosophies because they felt that by staying closer to the soil and doing the more natural things, they would not need drugs, hospitals and possibly medical treatments or doctor' care. I am sure that certain types of people are attracted to farming and certain types of people are drawn to the mental side of life. The mental people do not have the inclination to work with the soil like the physically-minded people do. There are many long-lived people among the Seventh Day Adventists, and they are a wonderful group of people. They balance their lives from a physical, mental and spiritual standpoint, especially those who closely follow Ellen G. White's work as given in the beginning. I consider her "Ministry of Healing" one of the finest books in my library.

DOUKHOBOR

Another group of people who I consider the finest I have ever met are called the Doukhobors. They are a group of people who emigrated from Russia to Canada many years ago. At one time they refused to follow the regime of the revolutionaries by becoming involved in their wars.

Some 1,500 of them migrated to Canada and settled mostly in British Columbia, drawing upon the royalties from the book called "Resurrection" written by Leo Tolstory for their travel needs. The Quakers were also instrumental in helping them to settle there. Mr. Peter Maloff, a Doukhobor, traveled with me in Russia, the country where his parents were born and raised. Russia still has people who live long lives and have a strong calcium in heritance in their bodies. This was demonstrated by the fact that they were willing to leave everything and come to Canada to take up working with the soil. They recognized that agriculture was of prime importance, and that it would take a lot of physical energy to do this. But nothing daunted them, nothing scared them. They were fearless in establishing themselves in a new and strange land. This takes a lot of calcium. This takes a good inheritance.

I have lived with these people and associated with them for more than 40 years, and I have found them to be the finest group of people I have ever met. They are true, honest, upright and solid; and I can say this about most of them, especially those I have met.

They went through hardships to begin with, but being men of the soil, and having a spiritual philosophy, they went ahead undaunted to accomplish things, and they stuck to their original beliefs. They are against war and I don't know of anyone who shouldn't be against war. They are peace-loving and they are people who would like to live in harmony. They are people who share their knowledge and who give of what they have; and they demonstrated this so beautifully when we needed work done on our Ranch. For instance, we needed a little gymnasium and we needed a dining room addition. They came in a group, fifteen at a time, to help build these for us. This was done without compensation, except possibly they realized that our teachings had helped them and they wanted to help us in return.

When you read some of their history, you can see that they were hard pressed. To begin with, they put as many as thirty women out to plow and take care of the fields while their men worked on the railroads. They started with just plain ground and built their own little communities. They had a wonder leader, Peter V. Verigin, a man who was aggressive and who had the acuity and spiritual knowledge for good leadership. He was one who believed in the natural life; he believed that by living close to the soil, you could develop a good body. He showed the others that having good foods, having a good larder with natural foods in the pantry, was the beginning of good health. He was a wise man, and I think a lot wiser than many of his own people realized. The ideals he upheld are an aid to living a long life, in good health. When I study these people I see that they are tillers of the soil, and they have more elderly people than any other group I know. I believe this is because they are hard workers, they don't believe in retiring, and they are people who are certain that the natural life was meant to be lived by everyone. They have integrated themselves into the Canadian influences, and we find that they are amenable to all things that are good. While they did not believe in many of the principles that man lays down in his laws, especially those that have to do with war and the education given to children, they still held to principles that fostered harmony and the very finest outlook and future for their children in their communities.

They are a religious people. The word, "Doukhobor", means "spirit wrestler" and they do wrestle with the spirit in trying to bring about the best for everyone in their community and all those who live around them.

Much of their history is unrecorded, but they remember it in their songs. Anyone who has heard the Doukhobor choirs will agree they are intensely moving because they recount their history and show their poignant feeling in what they have to bring forth to the world in general.

Originally, they sprang from a dissident group in Russia, that in the very beginning, sought the peace and harmony which they felt the world should have. They truly have wonderful Christian principles, for they feel that to kill any man is to be contemptuous of the will of God.

This sect is made up of various groups from different parts of Russia who have come together into the settlements. At one time they owned guns, knives and swords to fight with; however, they put them into a pile, poured kerosene over them and started a bonfire. They wanted nothing to do with war or any of the implements of war. In Russia, they were persecuted harshly, and their communities were pillaged causing them to seek refuge in other areas of the country. After many had died, a solution was worked out whereby they were permitted to leave the country in the year 1898. This was accomplished through the Society of Friends in England and through Tolstoy's efforts. They had to pay their own expenses and work out their own arrangements promising never to return.

The Canadian government was very aware of this group of people and finally accepted them, giving them land and exempting them from military service. It was here that they could live in harmony with the principles they held so dear.

While only 1,500 originally settled in the province of British Columbia, there are probably over 15,000 full-fledged Doukhobors at the present time.

In putting our Keys together, you will notice that we did not work with just the physical and mental but included the spiritual, as well. There are many precepts that people should live by, and we find that the Doukhobors believe that there are seven heavens to which man belongs and can strive for:

1. Humility
2. Understanding
3. Abstinence
4. Brotherly love
5. Compassion
6. Good counsel
7. Love

You can see that this takes in some of the Keys we have already discussed. The Doukhobors exemplified this list by being people of the earth. They truly are workers and tillers of the soil. They have very interesting ideas concerning the earth. They believe it belongs to God and not to any one man. It is the property of all mankind, and can be cultivated by everyone.

While they have had their problems and troubles in getting started, it is the same with all idealistic endeavors. Ideals have difficulty being expressed by the average person who is not educated or who doesn't have the same idealism as others. There are differences of opinion. Those who follow the soil and so not have a spiritual background or interest in spiritual things, are more inclined to get along better with each other.

The Doukhobors may have internal dissension and differences of opinion, but these are being worked out as they go along. In the refining process I do hope they come to a place where they can be the influence they would like to be for the rest of the world in their way of life.

In their work they take in the physical, mental and spiritual Keys that can give them a long life and good health. I have met many, many of these people who have lived a hard life but a good one, and they have enjoyed a healthy and a long life, as well.

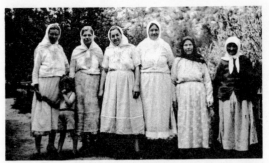

Representing three generations of the Maloff family—all vegetarians.

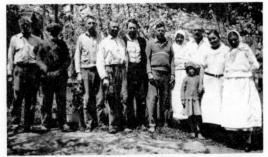

Hard working Doukhobors—tillers of the soil.

This is a typical house on the Kootenay River in surroundings where gardens supported and fed these people. This was the family home of the first Maloffs coming to settle in British Columbia.

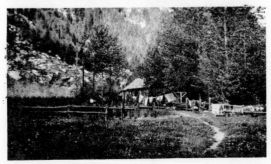

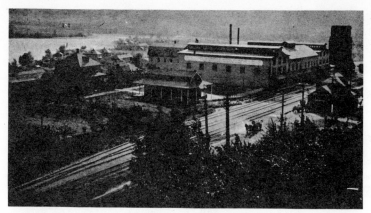

A large jam factory built in the Kootneays by the Doukhobors. A commercial venture that helped support them.

Group of Doukhobors from British Columbia who came to Hidden Valley Health Ranch to construct an exercise room.

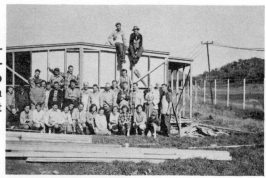

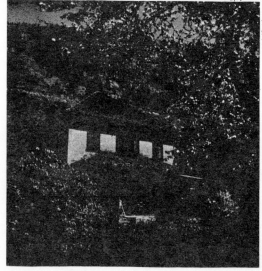

A typical two-story community residence that usually housed four families.

Chapter 9

Goat Milk—A Health Builder

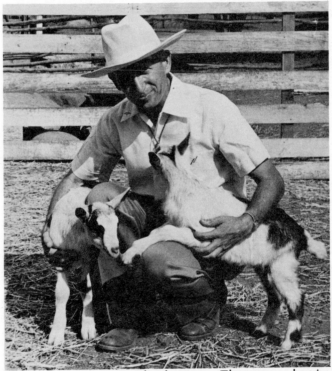

Wherever you go you find goats. They may be in the minority, but there isn't a section of the country I have visited where I haven't found someone who has a goat, and the reason for having one is for health. Everyone we visit has either had a child who was very sick and needed that type of milk to get well, or they had had a child who at one time was very sick, and they now use goat milk because they find it is the best.

For young and old alike, it has proved to be the one food that stays on the most unruly stomach. The most sensitive tissues seem to welcome the administration of goat milk in the diet. The sensitive stomach can use the high sodium content of goat milk. A broken down liver can handle the natural homogenized fat globules in goat milk. The fat cells being five times smaller in goat milk than in cow's milk, gives the liver an easier chance to handle this fat.

The high fluorine content, which is the beauty element and the one element which gives the teeth their hard coating and keeps the teeth from decaying, is found in the highest content in raw goat milk. It is ten times richer than in cow milk. Fluorine is that element which is like a volatile gas which leaves the milk when any heat has been applied. This is one of the reasons pasteurized milk is not good for human consumption.

We are getting a chemically unbalanced milk when we don't get all the elements that the milk originally had. Stomach ailments respond in a short period of time with goat milk and carrot juice. The most sensitive stomachs and the weakest bodies thrive on this diet. Arthritis, rheumatism and any of our acid conditions are helped when the health of the body has been developed through the use of goat milk.

Soaked and peeled dates with goat milk is a wonderful combination for ulcers of the stomach. Black mission figs and goat milk seem to set well and help those with arthritis.

Goat milk digests in twenty minutes while it takes two hours for cow's milk to digest. It is surely a vitality-producing food. Three-fifths of the world today lives on goat milk and thrives on it. It is one of the great things to sweeten the intestinal tract and to get rid of constipation. To develop a sweet intestinal flora use goat whey. This we can drink along with pineapple juice or any other sweet fruit juices.

At the Health Ranch we have administered goat whey enemas which have helped many extreme gas cases.

Goat milk is the best milk for feeding the baby. It compares in chemical balance so much to mother's milk. It has a chemical balance to feed goat kids which have more the structure of a human baby than does the calf. The calf has so much hide, hair and hooves to feed that the chemical balance in the milk is not as good for the human being as the chemical balance in goat milk. When man-made formulas do not work for the baby, try goat milk.

Loss of weight can be stopped by using goat milk and dried stewed fruits between meals. Using goat whey or skimmed milk will help those who want to reduce. Goat milk is alkaline in reaction because of its high sodium, potassium and calcium content. These chemical salts are so necessary in the human makeup. Because the goat is so fond of bark on trees and herbs and is really more of a browser than a grazer, we find the milk is high in silicone. This is one of the elements that is such an enemy of tuberculosis. We never find tuberculosis in goats or in goat milk while it is often found in cows.

While all milk is low in iron, we find that an addition of one or two tablespoons of blackstrap molasses to the milk we drink will help us in eliminating anemia. For the run-down condition, and when a life is dependent on the most easily-digested food, it is best to use warm goat milk directly from the goat. The animal energy and the heat seem to have a life-giving force that should not be overlooked. In our Health Ranch, we have practically seen the dead raised through the administration of warm goat milk in the last stages of most any disease.

GOATS WERE HIS LIFE

The story of George Surdel who lived on nothing but goat milk for more than 30 years, is an example of what goat milk can do if given an opportunity.

Goat milk saved his life in 1928 when he was near death in the mining town of Christopher, Illinois. He was seriously crushed by a rock fall when he was working in the New North Mine.

"The doctors patched me up, but I couldn't get my health back," Surdel said. "Then a friend told me about goat's milk. I tried it and my health miraculously returned."

After that he decided to gather a few goats. He soon had more than 40 of the animals—billy goats, nannies, and kids. George took good care of his goats. He led them to a grazing area every day. Each night he rounded up the stray kids and returned them to their mothers.

For breakfast, Surdel would have a cup of warm goat's milk. At lunch time, he'd go out and milk another goat. In the evening, it was the same thing. He lived on nothing but milk from his goats.

Although Surdel had been a soldier in World War I before becoming a miner, he refused a veteran's pension. He also turned down Social Security. "I don't need anything from anybody," he said. "My goats take care of me in winter and in summer. They're my life. I don't need anything else."

George Surdel had forty-two goats and perfect health. They went together.

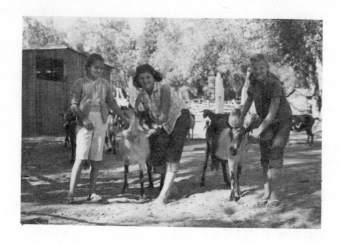

Chapter 10

Healing Powers
of Cabbage

In my travels to meet the elderly people, I found in Russia and Turkey especially, that there was a good deal of cabbage consumed. Every morning truckloads of cabbage were delivered to the Moscow markets. Of course, most people know that the basis for one of their national soups, borsch, uses mainly cabbage.

Some years ago there was a doctor who worked out experiments with raw juices and found that cabbage juice was one of the greatest juices for ulcers of the stomach. In fact, his experiments showed that within four or five days usage the pains in the stomach had ceased and the symptoms had disappeared. After this routine was followed for some weeks, x-rays showed that the ulcers had completely disappeared.

outside leaves contain 40 % more calcium than the inside leaves. If you will look at a cabbage, that extreme green is due to the heavy amount of chlorophyll that is in these leaves. Chlorophyll, of course, is one of the great healers in our bodies.

Examinations have shown that there is a healing power in the cabbage, and we have found from the study of our food history that the outside leaves contain 40 % more calcium than the inside leaves. If you will look at a cabbage, that dark green is due to the heavy amount of chlorophyll that is in these leaves. Chlorophyll, of course, is one of the most active healers in our bodies.

In Russia they claim that a good deal of benefit comes from cabbage, and that Vitamin C is very effective in chronic colitis, gastritis, and other organs of the body, including the liver.

We find a good deal of Vitamin C in the cabbage, and it is a preventive vitamin in resisting colds and all catarrhal conditions of the body which can be the basis of bronchial troubles, flu, etc.

The highest content of Vitamin C is found in the ordinary head of cabbage and today we are even able to find this Vitamin C manufactured in vegetable juice tablets. However, we believe that the fresh cabbage juice is the best way to take it.

Investigations have proven that there is as much Vitamin C in cabbage leaves as in lemons and in oranges. In cauliflower leaves we have even twice as much. This Vitamin C doesn't seem to be distributed throughout the cabbage texture evenly. The distribution is about 31½ % and the middle core contains as much as 71½ milligrams. Sauerkraut is so good because they use the central part of the cabbage. It is hard to believe but it is even claimed today that in the cooked state, cabbage has more available Vitamin C for the body than in the raw state. Most foods lose the Vitamin C in the cooking process.

Canadian scientists have found that Russian cabbage soup has more Vitamin C cooked, than in a raw condition. The cabbage juice, when it is boiled, received a third form of amino acids called "asckobigen". The release of this is one of the reasons that the cabbage is so good for the health of a person. There is also a lot of Vitamin A to be found in the outer leaves. Cabbage is also rich in phosphorus, potassium and sulphur.

In recent years, the Swiss have discovered a fermentative process with vegetables, and people are drinking a product called "Biota" which is obtained from health food stores. It is claimed that this ferment is exceptionally good for the intestinal tract. The cabbage ferment is found to have as many as 16 different amino acids.

Cabbage that is grated and strained through a cloth has more Vitamin C content than you can get through a common juicer. When cabbage has been stored in the root cellars and kept throughout the winter it seems to lose a certain amount of its Vitamin C content. It is well to know this fact—cabbage grown in the south is much richer in Vitamin C than cabbage grown in the northern regions. There may be a relationship between the carotene and the chlorophyll as it is brought to the plant life when grown in sunny regions.

I do believe that the leaves of all plant life are sunshine vegetables and carry this sunshine element for the control of calcium in the body. Much of my experiments and dieting procedures in the past have shown that ulcers of the leg, for instance, have improved best by using greens and the tops of vegetables.

In using cabbage juice for any particular purpose it is well to take it one hour before meals. It may be used three times a day. If we have a couple of glassfuls a day it would be a good quantity to overcome our condition, but to begin with, we might start with less. This is not always a pleasant-tasting juice for the average person. It is not to be taken until at least two hours after a meal, but it could also be used before meals. Using this therapy over a period of three to four weeks has brought wonderful results and is a great help for intestinal disorders.

Cabbage seems to be the poor man's vegetable. It gives the greatest return for the amount of work put into the soil and harvest. I am sure that the health of these long-lived people is due, in fact, to the large amount of cabbage they use in their daily diet.

Dr. Dean Burk spoke at a convention and told how years ago they had discovered certain properties in cabbages that had an anti-resistant value in the body, and that in the future there would probably be extracts from cabbage that could be used for many diseases in a natural way.

Dr. Burk has been the head of the cancer research institute in the Maryland hospital for some years.

Chapter 11

Running For Health

RUNNING IN NEW ZEALAND

While in New Zealand I became acquainted with a man by the name of Arthur Lydiard. He is a man who won the New Zealand Marathon in 1953, and also the Auckland Marathon in 1951. He is a great runner. He has inspired others to go into the running field, and it has produced many champions, one of the greatest being Peter Snell, who is our 1960 Olympic 800-meter champion and record holder.

In New Zealand a group gets together every once-in-a-while and its members have a good time just running off a lot of steam. They take a long leisurely run at about 6, 7, or 8 miles an hour...and they do this for their health. It has been found that these men become much healthier, more agile, more supple...their breathing capacity improves the oxygenation of the various tissues of their bodies.

We were with many of these people while in New Zealand. It is strange to see how they would go in for running as far as 20 to 25 miles each morning. Some of them do it only every Sunday morning. One of the men in the group, who had belonged to our Club in New Zealand, was a man 74 years of age. This man thinks nothing of running 20 miles in the morning before breakfast or before going to work. We visited a group that started out on a Sunday morning, some 40 to 60 of them, running throughout the countryside. They do this as a pleasurable jaunt. This has been carried on in this country, as Arthur Lydiard has been here and has started groups in some of our colleges.

Everyone seems to like to run. It appears to be part of a childhood fancy just to get out and run. I do believe that one of the most unusual things found in testing these men is the fact that they all seem to have a very slow pulse rate. Their hearts just pound away very slowly, but deeply and heavily. It was hard to believe that most of those I tested there, who had been running 25 miles each morning before breakfast, had a heartbeat that was averaging 40 beats a minute. This is considered very slow...on the other hand, they seem to develop a heart that is able to take care of their daily routine. To see these men of all ages capable of running this distance was very unusual. I do believe that the average person would be in better health if he did a little running exercise daily. It is one of the things that would keep him in fit condition. I was hoping that more colleges in this country would be taking this seriously now.

Arthur Lydiard has written a book called "Run To The Top", and anyone interested in running would certainly get an inspiration from reading his book.

RUNNING FOR FITNESS

At one time Arthur Lydiard did a considerable amount of football playing and entered into various sports. He thought he kept himself fit doing so, but one day he had an invitation to run with a man for over a distance of six miles. In spite of the fact that he thought he was fit, he was unable to run that six miles like the other man.

He made up his mind, at the age of 27, that if he could not run six miles like the other man, what would he be like at 47?

He started a physical training program of running, for he thought possibly that he could improve his bodily efforts and body tone and health if he would do some running.

He felt he had run too fast, and possibly more than his body could take in the beginning, so he started a program of a definite run each day. He did the job without anxiousness, and a great change was made in his running ability. He settled down to this daily routine and each day he grew stronger. Within a few months he was able to comfortably run miles each day without any disturbance in circulation or heart activity.

He found that an occasional extra effort in his exercise and running helped him to develop a little bit more fitness during the day; and he found that at times he could run 15 miles before work—work all day—and then run another five miles at night after working hours. His work did not suffer and he felt fit during the day.

He noted that in the beginning he had a pulse rate of 70 beats a minute, but it dropped steadily down below 60, and at times he found that his heartbeat would run 45 beats a minute.

This has been the most unusual aspect of my check-up of these men who do jogging. They have a very slow pulse beat which I think is conducive to living a longer life. Those who have a fast heartbeat wear out the heart.

Doctors have said that they believe that a half-hour of jogging is equal to at least two hours of any other exercise as far as general body toning and the efficiency of the cardio-respiratory system is concerned.

Arthur Lydiard has been running ever since the age of 27 and now in his 40's he still has a very slow pulse rate, his weight is trimmed down and his muscular development is quite youthful and supple. He also has the same drive and energy that he has had for many, many years.

I do believe that many people have gone to extremes in running and have caused some results that could be detrimental. But if it is done properly, and probably under a doctor's supervision, a person could develop a fit body through running.

One thing brought out in most of the runners is that they don't tire as much as they used to. They eat better, they sleep better and they enjoy life. I have talked to many who seemed to have worked out their problems better and especially so while they are running.

Arthur Lydiard brings out that fatty, starchy foods are not too good for the runner. He believes that for health we need good, wholesome food.

I've seen thousands of people in New Zealand running the Arthur Lydiard style, and he has done more to bring back the Olympic and marathon running than anyone I know. He was the National Marathon Champion at 36. In fact, it was Arthur Lydiard who trained Ray Crockett for the marathon for nine months. When they entered the National Marathon it was won by Crockett, the student, and Lydiard, the master, came in second.

Those who have done any jogging find that their perspiration is quite odorous, but this, of course, is due to the toxic materials that are being eliminated from the body. I am convinced that the body is made fit when we move along the acids and the toxic material that have developed in the body. They have probably been put there from poor foods and the living conditions we have gone through in years past.

I believe that in running the average person will feel that his intestinal organs work better and the bowels are better; and this can be used for the prolongation of life and to keep one fit.

It was Nurmi who had a pulse rate of 42 beats a minute, and it was claimed that this contributed to his resultant success in the Olympic games. He represented Finland and was one of the greatest runners of our time.

I think one of the main advantages of jogging is that we are building our daily stamina. Of course, stamina is needed to carry on our work without being tired. I am convinced, from a cholosterol standpoint, that as the circulation of the blood is increased, and as a larger amount of water is used, and with the increased perspiration that takes place (or the elimination through the skin), the cholesterol in those who do any distance running will be reduced.

Running, no doubt, helps to improve a stagnant bloodstream. By toning the muscles, the circulatory system is kept in good order throughout the day. I hear from the joggers that their mental keenness and alertness is always better, and this is of great value.

I am sure that the blood cells, as they pass throughout the body more quickly, carry a greater amount of iron and oxygen to do a better repair job so that more regeneration can take place. When we stop and think about the fact that the body is made up of some 80% muscle structure, it is well that we keep it in good order. I used to spend considerable time with Bernarr McFadden, and he would say that if you can keep your muscles fit, you can keep in good health.

It is through the muscle structure that we keep the circulation of blood traveling at a good rate. All the elimination in the body depends on the circulation. We depend on the circulation of blood to our glands for the youth of our glandular structure. It is a matter of keeping the body fit in any physical exercise possible. McFadden was a great advocate of cross-country walking and country-walking marathons.

As we continue with our research into running we find

that Larry Lewis would run 5 to 6 miles before breakfast. In fact, at the age of 106, I asked him to what he attributed his long life and he said, "Running before breakfast and drinking lots of water." I believe that this is a great factor to consider, because in keeping fit we have to have a good circulation and a good muscular working system.

While most of the runners I have checked into have no definite diet, we find that they did have a lot of fruits and vegetables and many of them had lean meat; but they usually gave up the real heavy foods as it seemed to make them logy and interfered with their running.

I have often said the beginning of all disease is the wearing of clothes. This is one of the first things we notice about joggers: they perspire well, they get their bodies out in the air, and they start a resistance program to the elements; and I feel this develops fitness and helps to develop that prolongation of life. I am sure this will be proven in the future.

One of the secrets of running is the fact that it is not a matter of seeing how far a person can run or actually building up the strength of the muscles; but it's a matter of building up the strength of the heart muscle, the arteries and the veins, and having that contractability develop, to keep the circulation in good order, and in this way be able to build a great stamina. It is the stamina that wins the game. I am sure that it is the stamina that carries on the life force in the body.

It was Bill Bowerman who did a good deal to build up the basketball team in Portland, Oregon. He was quite an advocate of Arthur Lydiard's system of jogging and started with an 8-minute-mile pace which the team was to hold for 15 minutes. He found that they were completely exhausted in 10 minutes time and couldn't continue. The next day most of the men did not come back, although he was able to get them together later on. In two weeks time, all the candidates could hold an 8-minute-mile pace for 45 minutes. This was developed through the jogging routine. I have seen the results of many joggers who had troubles with indigestion and many diseases which have been overcome through running. I do believe exercise is one of the necessary keys in having a good, fit body.

Some time ago I met Dr. Harold Elrick of San Diego. He is one who has stuck to the jogging routine and believed in exercising to balance the daily routine that the average businessman has created. Investigation and research has been done by Dr. Elrick on some of the runners; and a while ago he investigated the Tarahumarans, the foot runners, who live at the 9,300-foot level in the Sierra Madres. These tribes do a lot of distance running in the mountains of Chihuahua in Mexico, 300 miles south of El Paso, Texas.

These runners make a game of this by kicking a wooden ball while jogging. The teams have to go quite a distance to the finish line, so many times these games last up to three days. Of course, these days, we find much disease has come to these people and possibly there has been a change from life as it was in the past. The runners in New Mexico and in various parts of the world did unbelievable distance running because they kept it up day after day and kept their bodies fit.

Dave Powers is a personal friend of mine, and while he is 84 years of age at the present time, when I met him over 40 years ago, he was broken down in health. We helped him to start an exercise program and a correct-eating regimen. Through this diet, and starting a program of cross-country running and walking, this man broke four records. He still holds two of the records today in spite of the fact that at the time he was nearly 50 years of age. There were many younger men—25, 26, 27 years of age who were not able to keep up with him. Some of these records are unbroken up to this date.

RUNNING FOR HEALTH

By B. Barinov (of Russia)

Jack London in his Journey on the Snark tells of a very unusual self-recovery from a malady of a school teacher by the name of Ernst Darling from the state of Oregon. He was close to death, his weight had gone down to eighty pounds and he was so weak that he even was unable to talk. Doctors gave up hope and resigned. Then he re-solved, using his will power, that he must rebuild his life anew, and he did. The end of this documentary episode is so significant that Jack London has made an appeal to his hero: "I even now see you dancing and somersaulting on the deck. Your hair is in salt water, your eyes glittering, body a golden color from the sunshine. This recuperation is evident, activity, and activity."

Similar to this, but perhaps less exotic, an event has taken place with a man of our time, Mr. K. G. Solodov who, in his sixtieth year, suffered a heart attack. Three years of medical care gave no results; for 11 months the hospital bed tortured his nerves beyond any further endurance. Doctor's orders were always the same—rest, complete rest. They would not even allow him to walk on a level spot. He was really conscious of his end. And then at this visible crossroad, Mr. Solodov said to himself, "I don't want to die, and I am not going to die!"

Recently, on one of these beautiful, sunny autumn days, I found Mr. Solodov at the Textile Sport Stadium. He had already finished running several rounds of the field and was now playing volley ball. I saw in him a healthy athlete, bubbling with energy and happiness. He had just celebrated his 70th birthday, and what happened to him ten years ago is remembered only as an improbable and unlikely dream.

Yes, he saved himself by running, that slow, lingering run, which turned out to be a blessed savior for his whole organism. Mr. Solodov started by first running only a few steps at a very careful trot, and of course, closely listening to his own heart. Then he increased his running steps to 20, then more and more until he started to gradually run not only one kilometer, but increased this run daily to six kilometers. Of course these running sprints were not performed irresponsibly; Mr. Solodov prepared himself with all consideration and study. During this period he studied all medical and sport building literature on the subject. He also started to see the doctors specializing in sport health-building programs, and he never missed a chance to see and talk to all well-informed folks from whatever walk of life they came. He made his own analysis and at times took this report to his doctor. But Mr. Solodov did not follow all of the instructions and suggestions that were given him. He really has worked out his own program.

Now he is following this program for all time—one regime. As soon as he awakens, he begins to bring his whole organism into life. He takes 6 deep breaths, gives out eight short exhalations, and continues this technique for a while. Then he performs a series of exercises for the feet, stomach, chest and arms, etc. Finally, he does some bicycle exercises. He says, "Now, when I am ready to get out of bed, then I am ready to give myself a full charge of activity, and I begin my full run at the open stadium. I love weather, even at 4:00 am. If I go for mushroom gathering into the forest, I don't care if it is 13 below zero. I go for a run. All this program is finished in 40 minutes, including my morning cold rub."

Mr. Solodov also is fond of ski running. He can easily perform a 25 kilometer run. He also loves to skate and play volley ball. In all of his health building activity, he has achieved a stabilized weight of 70 kilograms. He walks with grace. He sleeps well, his last cardiogram examination having shown no trace of any heart disturbance. This also can be said of another man who has been running practically all of his life—Mr. Roshov. At present, he generally makes 12 normal rounds of the stadium, and then he adds six more run-abouts before he stops for the day.

Naturally, the people of Ivanoskovis region all practice running therapy—not only the old folks go for the play, but many of the younger folks follow it diligently as well. Whenever you pass by, especially early in the morning, you can see a group of running people, and most of this group are doing it for their health's sake. They are organizing a series of running clubs here and there. So, it means that this running therapy has a future.

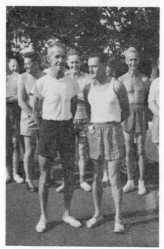

Right front: Arthur Lydiard, who has championed the jogging system throughout the world.

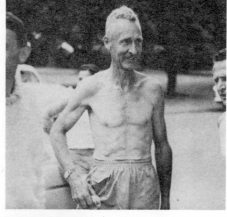

After 12 miles of running, Bill Meyer of New Zealand smiles happily.

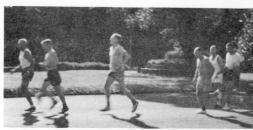

Jogging is popular throughout the world today because of Arthur Lydiard and his efforts.

Running is for all ages, but should be done under supervision.

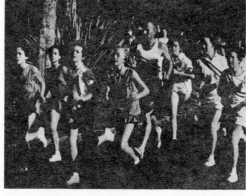

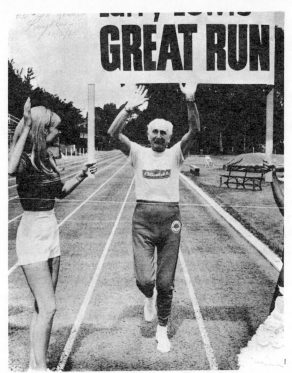

Larry Lewis, age 106, coming across the finish line in his running program.

Dave Powers, at age 82, still has unbeaten cross-country walking records that were set after a long period of much illness and return to good health.

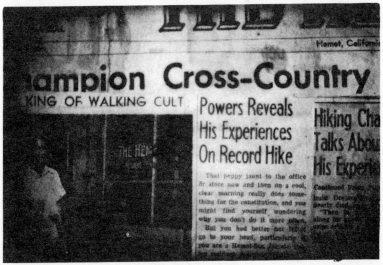

Chapter 12

Climate, Altitude and Air—Important Factors in Health

In regard to getting various people well, there are a lot of things that could be said about the various phases of the healing arts. If only we knew that certain types of people do better in one climate than in another, then possibly we would look into the climatic situation to find out what was needed—what it is in various climates that can give us better health. Many experiments have been performed to show that certain climates are better than others for our good health, and certain bodily conditions respond to our climate more than to another. Many experiments have been performed on rats and other animals to show that different altitudes and climates have definite effects on the lung structure, on the heart movement and on the water balance of the body.

For instance, with high blood pressure it is well to know that you cannot go to a high altitude, and sometimes a too dry climate is not good. We must consider how the patient will fare in a particular climate, altitude, temperature, humidity, etc.

FRESH AIR

There is a shortage of fresh air in all cities. Fresh air is best where trees are grown. The elderly always lived where there are lots of trees. They usually lived where there were a lot of pines. Pines throw off ozone better than any other tree. In fact, in Armenia, they call the pine the sacred tree.

Man cannot live without trees. Trees were considered the perfect symbol to follow among the Essenes. A tree was planted when a child was born in the Essene community. And a tree was planted every year of the child's life until he was 18, and then he was given a tract of land with the trees that were grown. This was his inheritance. We don't realize that trees are really an inheritance from God.

The old people lived where there was a multitude of trees. This brings the rain to them. You have heard of the rain forests? The rain comes because of these forests. It brings a humidity out of the clouds and atmosphere you don't get any other way. It doesn't rain in the desert much. The dust bowl doesn't have rain. If it was planted with trees, you would have rain there. We have the proper rain to keep things green wherever there are a lot of trees.

At the altitude of 4,000-7,000 feet pine trees will grow. It is hard for pine trees to grow near the ocean, but they grow at that altitude best. There is an extreme change of motion in air going from 4,000 to 7,000 feet. If you will notice it here, you will see that there is quite an exchange of the air right above our ranch located in the hills of Escondido. In the desert, it gets stagnant. The air becomes stale, but here, the cold of the ocean and the heat of the desert meet. We are right between. It is the heat of the desert that brings the cold air into the desert. This is why we have that extreme motion of air here.

If you want good water, get running water, moving water. If you want to get well, stay in air that is moving and passing by you quickly. It motivates good health in the tissues of your body. Metabolism is quickened, the thyroid works faster and you need to have this done as you grow older because the heart gets slower, circulation gets slower, and the skin responds less. Elimination is much better in a higher altitude, a rarefied air, drier air. In fact, all processes in the body, and especially elimination, are better as you go to a higher altitude. Climate, altitude, humidity, are some of the great keys we found with the elderly people.

THE AIR WE BREATHE

The air is composed of one part oxygen and four parts of nitrogen. There is a 1% gas called argon...also a small percentage of neon, krypton, and xenon. Oxygen is contained in our air by quantity close to 21%. (About 11 to 14 times as much oxygen in the air as usual would kill everything that lives. The death point in people is reached when the oxygen in the blood has been increased to about 34 percent by volume. If the oxygen is increased very slightly we do not thrive so well.) Nitrogen exists in our air to the amount of a little more than 78 %. Of course, the air can contain dust, insect wings, gases, water vapors, smoke, coal tar, fumes, ammonia, ozone, nitrous acid, sulphurous acid, sulphuric acid, nitric acid, bacteria, earth gases, bacterial gases, disease fumes, perfumes, odors, and other impurities.

Oxygen, when inhaled into the lungs, is attracted by the hemoglobin of the red corpuscles of the blood and carried by the circulating life liquid, the blood, into every organ, tissue, fiber and cell for purposes of oxidation. The hemoglobin in the red corpuscles of the blood contains iron which attracts oxygen. Blood carries carbon dioxide from the tissues to the lungs where the carbon dioxide is extracted and sent out into the air through the nose, which in one sense is a carbonic acid chimney. When the breathing function is not efficiently developed, the carbon dioxide in the tissues and blood is not carried away. This results in bloating and an acid blood and carbonosis, causing gas generation, gastritis and carbon dioxide symptoms. This is why it is necessary to breathe vigorously in high altitudes, together with the exercising of the muscular tissue in vital organs. Chest culture and muscle culture always favor health. However, breathing exercises we take are of no avail in getting the oxygen supply into our bodies many times, because we are lacking iron in the blood and in the tissues. It is usually the mental workers who suffer from oxygen deficiency. They need extra nerve fats, phosphorus foods and physical exercises.

A man at rest uses about 580 to 1,000 liters of air. A man doing physical work uses more than 1,000 liters in 24 hours...if he weights 250 to 300 pounds. A brain worker who uses only about 400 liters of air each day will soon suffer from bad blood, gas, acidity, bloating, brain fag and sleeplessness. Venous blood contains about 8 volumes less of oxygen than arterial blood...or 12 volumes of oxygen in one hundred volumes of blood; and 7 volumes more of carbon dioxide than arterial blood.

Respiration can vary from 3 breaths a minute to 30 breaths a minute. The respiration can vary in the same man at different times according to his state of health, development of the chest, brain, presence of gases in the system, the amount of food in the stomach, the degree of physical and mental depression, the condition of the lungs, state of mind, and size of chest, also his disposition, intensity of emotion, work, sleep, age, activity and many other conditions. The more powerful the lungs, the more reposeful the individual and the less number of breaths each minute. But the weaker the man and the more emotional, mental, nervous, and sensitive he is, the greater the number of breaths each minute.

We know that the air in an unventilated room is unfit for breathing. But did you know that those who have a lot of sugar, starch, and fat in their bodies produce more carbon dioxide in the blood and tissues and therefore need more oxygen? The more carbohydrate foods we eat, the more carbonic acid gas we make. The choke-gas does not allow the proper amount of oxygenation to take place in our bodies. Eventually oxygen hunger develops and diseases result. When we need more oxygen in the body, it is well that we learn to leave sugars, starches and fats alone and seek a higher altitude with dry air.

Without air, light, heat, moisture and plants as manufacturers of our foods, animals would not exist very long. We should realize that the plant kingdom—the vegetable kingdom—is a manufacturing concern which gives us a new supply of oxygen; and that men, birds and animals would soon breathe their last breath if it were not for the oxygen supply of the vegetable kingdom. Men, animals and birds thrive on oxygen while the plant kingdom thrives on carbon dioxide and nitrogen. Men, birds and animals utilize oxygen and exhale carbonic acid. Plants need carbon dioxide and nitrogen and give off oxygen for us to breathe. Here we can see the wisdom of the great World Builder. The more abundant the garden around you, the more trees, plants and flowers, the more oxygen and ozone in the air. Wind and light help to purify the air and are therefore a great blessing to us. Carbon dioxide decreases as we ascend into high altitudes but increases enormously in crowded cities because of the many lungs, manufacturing plants, and lack of vegetable life.

Carbonic acid is more abundant close to water surfaces, but at higher elevation it decreases. There are some people who benefit by carbonic air and moisture while others improve in localities where carbon dioxide is minute in quantity, where the air is dry.

Air that contains 35 % carbonic acid gas paralyzes the lung centers and kills at once. A strong healthy man cannot live more than 5 minutes in such air. Carbon dioxide in excess in blood, stomach tissues, secretions and waste matter is one common cause of blood pressure, acid formation and gas generation. Odors can stimulate the lungs, brain, chest and vital faculties, the senses and the appetites. Dust is a vehicle of disease germs. It is usually the dust that carries deadly bacteria. The more dust in the atmosphere the more germs in the air. In a big, dusty city mouth breathers are never safe.

In analyzing the air, Ehrenberg found some 460 different organic substances in it. It's no wonder we are sick, taking in all the metal dust, smoke, chalk, clay, wood fibers, disease vapors, sand, scales, capsules, legs of insects, wings, vapors, odors and so forth. It is a wonder that we live at all, especially in the cities with the modern automobile and the lack of vegetation!

There is more carbon dioxide in the city than in the country. This is why city people always have more carbon dioxide in their systems. This leads to acidity, gas in the stomach, bloating, gastritis, rheumatism, stiffness, stomach trouble, headache, colds, catarrh, asthma, carbonosis, acidosis, etc.

Dr. Arthur Vos, MD, wrote: "Of all the food required by the body, 90 percent must be oxygen. A man weighing 150 pounds is composed of 110 pounds of oxygen by weight. If the oxygen contained in his body were set free, it is estimated that it would fill 750 cubic inches of space."
(Philosophy of Health)

Dr. E. E. Marin, MD, said: "Science tells us that over half of our maintenance comes in the air and oxygen we inhale. This means that pure air is much more important than the food we eat. We can live without food for 3 months without much inconvenience, but we can hardly live 1 minute without breathing."
(Truth Teller, January 1940)

Dr. Thomas Darlington, former health commissioner of New York City stated: "The products of combustion irritate the eyes, nose, throat, the respiratory tract, bronchial tubes, and gastro-intestinal area. In the lungs the carbon particles become imbedded in the air cells, and in time the lungs change in color from natural pink to black.

"I have performed many autopsies upon New Yorkers

and almost without exception their lungs were as black as night.

"There is a striking parallel between smokiness of cities and higher pneumonia mortality. The soot, having coated the interior of the lungs, obstructs their natural eliminative processes and the flow of oxygen into the blood." (Quoted by W. B. Courtney in "Our Smoky Cities," in Collier's.).

The press of March 6, 1944, reported that coal gas from the locomotive of a freight stalled in a tunnel in Italy killed 500 persons. Only 49 lived to be taken to hospital.

The hemoglobin of the blood has an affinity for carbon monoxide gas approximately 300 times greater than for oxygen. The air in the cities and on the highways where there is much traffic is so saturated with carbon monoxide gas, that the blood becomes only part oxygen-hemoglobin while the other part becomes carbon monoxide-hemoglobin. This lack of oxygen makes people pale, weak, anemic, dizzy—and they look to food for relief.

ELECTRICITY

Electricity is said to be one of the forces of Nature. In reality it is God at work in Nature. It is God's Power House. The positive and negative electricity is probably the male and female energy that is the essence of Cosmic Electricity or the vital force at work in earth and sky. The atmosphere is positively electrified. The Earth is negatively electrified. Negative and positive electricity cannot exist separately. The air is charged with electricity. There is more in the air in summer than in the winter; under the influence of heat, light and sunshine, the vegetable kingdom generates electricity. Electricity is converted into light and heat and motive power. When there is an increase of electricity, the principle of growth is at work constantly in men, animals, or vegetation. Forests cool the air and produce fog, clouds, and rain. This is why plans are being made to re-forest the Sahara Desert. It will attract water to this arid ground.

The less light the less plant growth. The less light the less oxygen and the more carbon dioxide in the body. Thunder storms are few in winter, but in the summer they are numerous. The less light the less electricity in the air.

The less light the less electricity in the air—and the more female trouble! Light in the oxygen makes the blood more alkaline by the removal of carbon dioxide. Light improves electrical generation in the muscles and electrical tensions in the atmosphere. Light has a chemical action upon nutritive function and plant life. To improve the nutritive function, light should be permitted to the body.

When we study climatology we are interested in the air chemistry: air pressure, winds, humidity, light and its influence, what ultraviolet effects we receive at one altitude and another, the temperatures and their effect upon the skin and the organic structure of the body, even the electrical effects. Those who are interested in health should recognize that what we eat and drink is a necessary part of health building, but also that the existing climatic phenomena can add to our health or take away from it.

We should know that the friction of clouds, winds, hail, evaporation, snow and changes in gases alter the electrical tension of the atmosphere and that this has a tremendous effect on the nerves, brain and blood of certain types of people. Many cannot sleep, they cannot recuperate properly when the electrical tension is high. In their restlessness you find them seeking another place to go for their vacation and for their good health. High-tensioned people should not seek the high tension electrical regions. High tension electricity with its great electrical variation is not always favorable to nerves, mind and the senses, especially of those people who are built upon the principle of intensity and who are inclined to develop fears easily.

During electrical storms ozone is formed. We notice this most as we go into the mountains after an electrical storm. The cerebellum, or chest brain, is stimulated in these ozone belts. Ozone is important to the consumptive and to certain highly-nervous people. Nervous distress is nearly always favored by a breezy climate, but oxygen must be in abundance in such a climate, and the muscular system must not be weak. Consumptives thrive in ozone belts. Many types of paralysis, hysteria, paralytic ailments, dropsy, anemia, lost manhood, mental depression, tired feelings and a weakened cerebellum improve in this belt. Ozone can be like a powerful tonic, however, and too much of it can weaken the body. Ozone in excess does harm to the blood and to the pulmonary circulation.

Mountains are wonderful for a vacation. They are usually full of pine odors, and have less carbon dioxide. People with a low breath capacity or consumption, and others, should go to a higher altitude where carbonic acid is less abundant. Invigorated, toned up to the point of friskiness, this is where we feel new. Mountains make an ideal vacation place. Night sweats usually disappear in the mountains. When the skin is always damp the vital organs are not protected. The system loses its heat. Health resorts owe their curative power to such agents as air, exposure to the sun, vigorous exercises, massage, ozone, climate, air pressure baths, light rays, altitude, rest, vegetable luxuriants, peace, change of habits, etc. When going on a vacation, consider the dust that is in the air, the manufacturing that is going on, the humidity, altitude, heat, cold, drafts, winds and air pressure.

AIR PRESSURE

A rise of temperature is known by a fall in the barometer. The presence of moisture in the air affects the barometer. Moist air is much heavier than dry air. The air pressure is not the same at different times of the day. It rises toward sunset; it usually falls as heat increases. Warm air expands and ascends, and cold air takes its place. This produces the air circulation or air motion called wind. Thus, air motion gives rise to wind. Land cools by radiation, and cold sea breezes cool the evenings. Sea breezes are cold air flowing from the sea to the heat absorbed land. This is why wind blows from the land toward the sea at night. Night wind is the opposite of day wind. Night wind is land wind. Day wind is sea wind. There is a constant interchange of sea air and land air day and night.

Storms are nothing but air in motion. When the wind blows at the rate of 3 miles an hour or less we call it a stand-still...a calm. When air moves 8 miles an hour the wind is hardly noticeable. When the air travels 13 miles an hour, we call it a pleasing breeze...16 to 19 miles an hour we call a gentle breeze at work. Air circulating 22 to 24 miles an hour is a moderate breeze; 27 to 29 miles an hour, we have a fresh breeze; 34 miles an hour, a medium wind. A gale is from 38 to 42 miles an hour. In a fresh wind, the air moves at 37 to 49 miles an hour. A strong wind travels 56 miles an hour. When the air moves at 64 to 68 miles an hour, we have a storm; and if it moves at 75 miles an hour, we call it a strong storm. In a hurricane the air travels 88 to 130 miles an hour.

Rain is man's best friend in the sense that it purifies the air...but it is his enemy because a storm increases germ life. Microbes increase enormously when it begins to dry after a rain. In dry weather great clouds of dust are found in the air. The better time to breathe freely is in the winter, spring, and after a rain.

Rain decreases inorganic substances in the air, but it increases micro-organisms almost unbelievably. Dust, dirt and impurities, however, are more dangerous than germ life. Pathogenic bacteria never stay long in the air because of light, rain and wind. Such bacteria are thrown to the ground by the rain. A salt moisture is found in the air to a certain extent...evaporated from the ocean, and it floats about as little salt globules and particles. A salty air has a soothing effect upon sleeplessness, nervousness, hysteria, temper and restlessness.

The weight of air is considerable when we realize that there is an air pressure of from 11 to 15 tons bearing down on us daily, yet no one is conscious of this tremendous load that presses upon him.

Gases expand upon heating and rise. Atmospheric pressure therefore diminishes in proportion as we ascend; the higher we go, the less pressure. The air is thinner, rarefied; the air molecules are farther apart. It is cooler because as gases expand, temperature drops. When we go into higher elevations we should ascend slowly, gradually.

ALTITUDE

In the Caucasus and in the Hunza valley where we found the oldest people, and down in Vilcabamba, the average altitude is from 4,000 to 7,000 feet. There is only about a 3,000 foot difference there, but this is the ideal altitude. There are many things to be said about this Key. As a person grows older, we find that he should be in a higher altitude. The reason for this is that our metabolism is faster and the thyroid works faster. If we get too high, the heart will have to work too fast and hard. Blood pressures can go up and we grow older if we go too high.

An altitude like we have at the Ranch is perfect as we

grow older. This is a lovely thing. I believe Escondido could be used as an example of a good place to grow old if a person would put all of these parts of health together. This is a great country. It has a 2,000 ft. altitude, with clear sunshine and pure air. If you put all of these things together you can actually see how we can have long-life people in a place like this.

As people go to a higher altitude, the blood count always gets higher. You need a high blood count in order to keep well and keep the body in good order. You cannot repair, rebuild, or replenish without a good high blood count. That is the secret of our work. You find as you go to the higher altitudes in the Andes, you can have a blood count as high as 7,500,000. The highest blood count you can get down at the ocean is 5,000,000, because of the pressure existing at a low altitude. In order to get well, the Good Book tells you to go to the mountains, go to the hills for your strength. Well, these old people were already living in the mountains. They didn't know they were already living in a perfect place. I interviewed Mr. Gasanov in Baku and his doctor was there. I asked the doctor what his blood count was, and it was 6,500,000. This is what kept that man well. It's something to think about, isn't it?

At sea level people are known to have about 5 million red blood corpuscles per cubic millimeter...but living in high altitudes of 5 to 6 thousand feet, the red corpuscles increase to 7, or even to 8 million per cubic millimeter, providing that high altitudes favor an increase in the red blood cells. In the mountains people have red blood corpuscles in greater numbers than they have in a lower altitude. For instance, in the Andes Mountains in South America, at some 10 to 12 thousand feet many people have blood counts of 7,500,000, an almost impossible blood count to obtain when living by the ocean. There may be much truth in the saying, "Go to the hills for thy strenth."

Divers and others who work in dense air suffer from anemic symptoms. They suffer from pain in the limbs, grow weak and become anemic. Oxygen under high air pressure becomes toxic, and the red blood disc decreases alarmingly. Mountain sicknesses, on the other hand, are peculiar to people who suddenly go to high elevations. At first our nervous system is irritated by high altitude—temper increases, we become more violent, fussy, morose; hunger and thirst increase. If the altitude is excessive to us, our digestive functions suffer. If, however, our vital functions can respond to the change of altitude, we soon feel as wonderful as if we were born anew, as if our lungs were lined with cotton. We become more active, our functions are sharpened, the brain is clearer. We think right, concentrate better, compose better poetry, feel more important, make greater inventions, accomplish greater deeds.

At a higher altitude and in a drier climate, we breathe entirely differently. We have a greater expansion of the chest; oxygenation takes place more rapidly, metabolism is quickened, and the thyroid gland works at a much more rapid pace.

If we go too high, however, new symptoms and ailments appear. Our red blood cells are the oxygen carriers in the body. Our lungs are actually an oxygen pantry where the red corpuscles go for their oxygen supply. The more red corpuscles we have, the more oxygen we can utilize. In a higher altitude we can become more irritable, impatient, impulsive, more thirsty and hungry, more urgent and imperative, more active in spirit, more willing to work, more inventive and less tired. In too high an altitude we can become dizzy, we can have a roaring in our ears, our senses can be impaired, our hearing become dull, vision dull, mind stupid; we get sleepy and sluggish, and we suffer from oxygen hunger.

Hens stop laying in high altitudes, however we feed them. Dogs do not breathe 13,000 to 16,000 feet above sea level. Trying to raise cats at an altitude of 14,000 feet will prove to you that there is a good lesson to learn in climatology. You cannot breed cats at that altitude. Muscular effort is nearly impossible. Unusually high elevations produce a high, nervous pulse and increase the number of respirations per minute to the point of fevered breathing. Nervousness is increased at a high altitude and decreased at a low altitude. Unusually high altitude produces a rapid pulse and a feverish respiration...makes the heart tumultuous and the breath as rapid as an intimidated bird...it makes all people nervous. Work that is easy at low altitudes for most people is difficult at a very high elevation. An excessive elevation may develop heart disease, lung trouble, especially hypertrophy of the heart, because thin air throws a greater strain on the right atrium of the heart, owing to the fact that the blood is not sufficiently charged with oxygen. This throws an extra strain upon the valves of the heart. Send a flesh-clogged or soggy, waterlogged lady or man to a high altitude, and they will both suffer from suffocation.

HUMIDITY

Humidity is the invisible water vapor in the air...not snow, fog, rain or dew. Relative humidity is the watery gas or vapor present in the air as compared to the vapors that it can hold. Cold air holds less humidity. The higher we go, the less humidity. The more the air expands, the less water vapor it can hold. Dry air has less water vapor. If air cools beyond its saturation point, precipitation results. Fogs are low clouds. Rain means greater condensation of water vapor in the air. Dew is deposited moisture. Hail is frozen raindrops, often strongly condensed. Ice is frozen water. Steam is watery evaporation by heat (or otherwise).

Dry air permits the sunbeams and light to pass through it. Moist air absorbs light, heat and sunshine. When moist air moves briskly and is cold, we lose heat so rapidly that the next day we are "under the weather" with a cold, and our nasal membranes are congested. A dry climate has many changes of temperature caused by the sun's heat in the daytime and the great heat radiation at night.

There is more heat where there is more vegetation, which is especially true around the equator. Vegetable exuberance moderates both heat and cold. Moisture intensifies both heat and cold, while dry air decreases heat.

Dry air makes tissues more alkaline than any diet. When the skin evaporation is poor. the kidneys are overworked. To improve the evaporation of the skin or quicken the skin function, aids the kidneys in times of kidney disease. When the skin is sluggish, the kidneys work double shift. A moist, warm, congenial climate relieves the kidneys, but a cold climate does not. An active skin relieves the kidneys. When we have a high or slightly high humidity, the skin function is always more active, as more water vapor is removed by the skin from the body. Evaporation of bodily heat decreases as the water vapors of the air increase; thus, we feel uncomfortable in warm, stuffy air. A high temperature and muggy air always lowers respiration and functional activities; it also increases the carbon dioxide in blood and tissue. In cold weather more carbon dioxide is exhaled and breathing has a wider, deeper range.

People whose internal heat is low have a very sluggish skin. This is why purification of the system falls so heavily upon the liver, lungs and kidneys. These organs become overworked and result in liver, kidney and lung diseases. Some 7 % to 8 % of the bodily heat is lost through the evaporation process performed by the lungs. Muscles are the great oxidizers and heat producers in the body. When the cerebellum is weak, we suffer from cold feet, hands, chilly sensations, colds, catarrh and perhaps pneumonia.

It is well that the heat generation in man be dissipated easily. More than 70 % of bodily heat radiates through the skin. If we did not radiate this heat continually, we would come to a boiling point and be cooked...in less than 40 hours. Excess body heat is lost through radiation, evaporation, perspiration and convection. At certain altitudes we find that this takes place better than at others.

The *humidity* that comes in the heat of the south keeps people perspiring so heavily that the sodium salts are lost through perspiration. Sodium salts are necessary in order to keep us young, and active, youthful, limber and pliable. Whenever we perspire too much, it takes the sodium salts from our joints and from the stomach wall. This is the reason women develop stomach and joint troubles during change of life. They are the ones who produce a "menopausal arthritis" because of constant sweating and the hot flashes. This is where they lose the sodium. Today, we take a gland food to overcome this when we find we need a lot of sodium at that time.

WHICH CLIMATE?

We should know that a cold bracing climate and a high altitude (that is, from 2,000 to 6,000 feet) tone our functions, increase appetites, build new red blood corpuscles, promote oxidation in the tissues and blood. However, in high altitudes our hearts must be sound.

Weak people, old people, lazy people, paralyzed people, thrive in a warm climate; but healthy people, people of high production, muscular people and great workers are comfortable in a cool climate. They become subject to infectious diseases in hot climates. Cold increases energy, but heat decreases it. Breathing is decreased in hot weather, and the removal of carbon dioxide is more difficult. People in hot climates are less energetic and more sociable. People in cold climates are greater fighters and less sociable. Cold winters lead to muscular action. Hot weather favors indolence. Moderate exercise of muscles and nerves and a breezy climate favor the element of the muscular and nervous systems.

Normal cold increases the elasticity of arteries and heart, but heat decreases these. People in a cold climate have a slower pulse and higher blood pressure. People in the tropics have a higher pulse and a lower blood pressure. Small size people have a quicker pulse than larger people. The skin pores are always active in hot climates, but they are sluggish in cold climates. Perspiration carries off heat and moisture through the skin in a hot climate.

Some people can withstand more heat than others. Dark-skinned people can endure it better than white because they have more nitrogen in the skin and less generation in muscular electricity. Every person, however, has less resistive power in the summer than in the winter. Our blood is always in a worse state in the summer than in the winter. Most germs die at 40 degrees below zero. Disease affects people differently at different seasons. Life is less productive in cold regions.

Temperatures affect the sex functions. Warmth develops sexuality unless heat is excessive. Heat increases the generative function. There is more sexual excess in hot climates than in cold climates. Sexuality is more active in a warmer climate. The menstrual function begins earlier in a hot climate. Child bearing is attended with greater difficulty in a hot climate because of a tendency to hemorrhages. Warmth develops the sexual system and increases sexual power.

Heating food, on the same principle, develops sexuality. Wind is bad for the sexual system and for people who suffer from sexual weaknesses.

Excessive heat destroys tissue as does excessive cold. Great heat makes the blood toxic and melts the myolin cells in spinal cord and brain. When the myolin cells melt, the man is in danger. This we call sunstroke. Sunstroke kills; excessive cold kills also. If the cold is excessive, all vital processes suffer, and unfavorable results follow.

Cold, as you know, constricts the surface blood vessels beneath the skin, lowers skin activity and the capillary function of the circulation so that the skin is not properly nourished. The skin is robbed of its fatty principle, sebum, and then it cracks and chilblains form. Wounds fail to heal because of lowered vitality and faulty circulation. Such a climate is too severe for our well-being. Regenerative functions suffer in a very cold and windy climate. Manhood is seldom at its best. Motherhood functions act under lower pressure, giving rise to menstrual difficulties and female ailments.

EXTREMES ARE DANGEROUS

Going to extremes in climate is always dangerous. It is not wise for anyone to change climate and stay for good. A man who goes from a hot climate to a cold climate and lives there the rest of his life may be healthy, but his offspring will suffer and die early. This holds good also for one who goes from a cold to a hot climate. A climate can be a tonic to one man, depressive to another, and even death to a third.

There are many books written on climate, but I think one of the nicest probably is the one by Clarence A. Mills, M.D., named, "Climate Makes the Man". He answers a good deal of the thoughts on what climate does to us. He is one of the leading men in the field of experimental medicine and has studied climate for many years. He shows where climate plays a dominating and startling role in all that we do. He shows that it affects our growth, speed of development, resistance to infection, fertility of mind and body, happiness, and length of life. He shows where it lulls the people of the tropics into passive complacency and drives those of the temperate zone into restless activity. He shows where sexual development is actually retarded by extremes of heat and cold. He has worked with many rats and mice and other animals and gathered together tremendous lots of valuable information. He even goes into showing the ideas of the varying effects of caffein, alcohol, and nicotine under different climatic conditions; shows where hardening of the arteries, tuberculosis, sinusitis and many ills are related to man-made weather, air conditioning, etc. He also points out that different diseases are related to various types of weather.

For instance, in some of his work he shows that breeders of small animals around Cincinnati frequently find that their charges are almost completely sterile by the end of a hot summer, while the same rabbits, mice or guinea pigs can, in cool winter, continue to reproduce profusely. One beautiful male rabbit, known to be highly fertile, was overheated in their laboratory hot-room but recovered to apparent good health; afterwards, repeated mating showed him to be permanently sterile. In Panama's warmth the prolific guinea pig becomes a poor breeder, improving slightly during the short dry season when low humidity renders the warmth less depressive. Large numbers of guinea pigs are required for certain hospital and laboratory procedures in Panama, but those imported from the North endure the heat poorly and are of little value.

During the severe heat of the 1934 summer in the Middle West, fertility was sharply reduced. Kansas City showed a 30 % reduction in conception rate during the month when day temperatures rose above 100 degrees. The usual summer decline is only 15 % . All through the Middle West birth certificate statistics showed the same sharp decline for conception during that period of the blazing heat.

Dr. Mill's advice to some of his patients in cases of sinusitis and high blood pressure is to seek a warmer climate. In another case, he tells one of his patients with high blook pressure to leave Wyoming, where he was trying to get well, and seek the relaxing warmth of southern Florida. He says that most physicians in the tropics now appreciate the importance of lowered virility in hot climates and send their patients out to more invigorating regions as soon as tuberculosis is detected. But the wise doctor will take care that his move does not plunge his patient into the respiratory hazards of winter cold and storms. Here again, the dry non-stormy southwest offers the region of choice.

Dr Mills has shown that the blood pressure of an American usually falls during a few year's stay in Peking, and that of a Chinese rises when he comes to the northern United States—even without any change in dietary or living habits. He tells of two of his Peking faculty colleagues, both native Britishers, experiencing a 30 % fall in blood pressure within a year after returning to China from furloughs spent in England or the U.S. In Peking it was difficult to find enough cases of hypertension—high blood pressure—for teaching purposes. While in Cincinnati, almost a third of the hospital beds were occupied by this type of patient.

So it is easy to see that temperature, altitude, humidity, winds and electrical differences in the atmosphere can have quite profound effects upon us, and especially in disease—these must be taken into account.

Chapter 13

Philosophy

Philosophy is an important subject to consider in the program of building a long life, for it is in philosophy that we use the mind properly and use faculties that we love to use, or we are constantly in disturbances that break down the mental faculties. Each person is built differently and each brain is built differently. Some are born geniuses in certain directions—some have talents that are lying latent, not even being used. Many times it is necessary to recognize that each person is different and works differently under particular circumstances.

Through our experiences we develop a philosophy. Many times it has been said that a man has to get his ears knocked down before he starts on a new path and follows the way that is good for him to pursue. It takes a certain mind and a very comprehensive philosophy for the writer to weave his story and put it on paper, or for the businessman to explain the manifold uses of his tools, instruments, utensils and apparatus that he sells. The lawyer has to understand the connection, and the bearing of cases presented to him so that he can clear up the important points. The organizer has to plan; the construction man has to have an organization that many times is highly complex. Yet all of this can be done, for there are mental faculties that can accomplish these things well. There are structural senses, and there are people who love to build—people who are interested in molecules and atoms and the far-out things that the average person wouldn't even think about.

We have people who are interested in manufacturing. There are some people interested in mechanics, who have a technical skill and a creative aptitude along this line. Some people have an inborn knowledge to know just how to take up a new subject. Some people are very practical, some people are very aesthetic, and all of this helps to develop a different type of philosophy as we go from one thing to another. Some people are not able to concentrate as well as others. Some can remember what they see well; others can remember only what they hear well. Some people live in their imaginations. Some people are very superficial in what they are doing, while others are truth-loving and often deeply spiritual. Some are inventive, and some are very thoughtful; they think things over. Some people live in mental pictures and they live in mental photography. Some are very exacting and do not create. Some people hold things in thought a long time and others can get things off their minds quickly.

For one person to say to another, "This is what I would do—why don't you do it this way," or, "Why don't you forget it," is not right. We find out that no two people are built alike and it is in this philosophy, especially as our civilization stands today, that we have to take care of the complex activities that are around us. The person who is extremely spiritual and is interested in the saints of the past, will talk about the love of those saints; and he will give you an aesthetic viewpoint that no man can give you who is interested in steel, iron, or mundane things.

We need to understand the general principle that holds this philosophy together in a united whole. It is a plan which permits all parts to act in harmony one with another. It is well to be able to see in philosophy that there is a connection and a unity in all the operations of nature, whether it includes the planetary bodies revolving in limitless space, the chlorophyll in parsley, or the living soil. Each has its own place, but each is part of the whole.

Very few people can go through life and have a philosophy that takes in everything: the structure of cloth, the tissue of man, the composition of stone and metals, the fossils and matter in general. Very few can examine from various viewpoints the quality, organization, compactness, density, or rarity of different materials. Very few can visualize in their minds how they can annex, establish, add on to, or rearrange objects or buildings. Some do very well in the literary field and are thoroughly versed in grammar; others will study all their lives and never grasp the language as well as they should. "As a man thinketh," they say, "so is he." Some that may seem unschooled or illiterate could be experts in a certain direction. At least they could be handy and have an aptitude with their hands that the man with a keen intellect may not possess.

So we have great skills inherent in our minds, and as we

ponder this we see that we develop a philosophy according to the mental faculties we have. We have to recognize how to combine and unify these faculties in order to make our thinking fruitful, otherwise we become one-sided. We bring things to a point without seeing the whole.

Many people are destructive in nature because they do not have enough love in their hearts. They may be sadistic and others may die as a result of their treatment, not able to bear these trials. This tendency may have to change; we may have to develop a love and understanding in its place. I hear this constantly from my patients, "If he only understood me..." "If he could only take more time to realize who I really am..." "We have no real communication..."

It is necessary that we study the functional and operative activities of the different parts of the brain, as well as their relationship with each other. We have to realize that in these functions we live our lives, and that we must go through life knowing we cannot live without this brain. The soul lives in matter and thinks through matter in the brain. It is not the brain that thinks, for when the soul departs, the brain and body function no more. The body is dead; the brain cannot produce one single thought, nor can the liver secrete bile, nor can the heart pump the blood. Many of us do not realize that there is more to this body than just the physical, just bones, just a hank of hair. There is more to this body than just the mental faculties of the brain. There is the soul that we have to consider. Some go deeply into this philosophy and have much to say about it, others only condemn because they do not investigate and know what is brought out in other people. To condemn before you investigate something is certainly criminal.

I am convinced that many people have educated themselves beyond the level of the average person. You can study to the point where people won't understand what you are talking about. We have added material here about music and color; and to the person who doesn't understand music, or who doesn't have a deep feel for what colors do for us, or whose aesthetic senses are not properly developed, you will find that such a person will not know just what is going on. He will be left behind, so it is well to recognize that study and philosophy are two of the greatest things we have in the development of mankind.

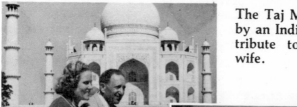

The Taj Majal was built by an Indian Prince as a tribute to his beloved wife.

The basis of Sai Baba's teaching is to bring love among all people and countries.

When a man has a philosophy that includes love, it also includes philanthropy, it includes understanding, sharing, peace and harmony—and he is able to put all of these things together—then that man is going to give his body the best care possible. I am convinced that the mind faculties, and the way you think, are going to express themselves in every cell of the body, and every physical movement will be felt by the brain activities and by the motor activities of the brain cells. Every nerve has its ultimate reaction in the muscle structure, in your digestion, in your breathing. If we recognize that there is a direct relation between taking care of our minds from a physical standpoint so that the physical body can be taken care of, then we would realize that food has its place. We would realize that altitude can affect the nervous system. The altitude and climate together have a certain combination that we need. The Keys throughout this book are given to you in a general form; but if we could sit down and show you the relationship between one and the other, you would recognize that perspiration, acids in the body, the bone marrow in the body, the love of the mind, the philosophy we entertain, the tranquility of the scene around us, all contribute to either a long or a short life. The absence of disturbances lenthen it. It is the constant stirring around of aggravations that can kill us. We need a philosophy of life that will give us a long and healthy one.

Much could be said about philosophy, but it is the inner activity, the interplay of the whole body, that we have to consider. It is not just inheritance. A weak body, well-cared for, can live a long life. A person without calcium, even though he is born where there is a lot of calcium in the soil, is in trouble. If he is living on junk foods, foods that produce acids and break down the kidneys as well as other organs in the body, we find that philosophy will never do him any good. The frugal eater is probably the wisest person we have talked about, and temperance is probably the greatest Key of all. I am convinced that these people don't need much food to sustain the body; they don't need the stimulation that the average person thinks he requires today from his diet and foods. Temperate people have a philosophy that is good for their bodies—that does not tear them to pieces—and that allows them to repair and rebuild beautifully in their natural environment.

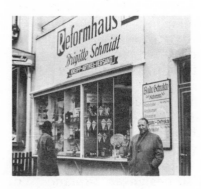

The Reform House. We may have to know where we can get the proper foods to rebuild our health. We may have to reform our ways.

God in his wisdom has given us foods from his garden which are wonderfully and fearfully made.

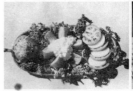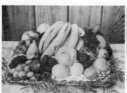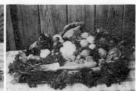

Foods I served at Hidden Valley Health Ranch can be found everywhere.

These elderly people don't even know that they were supposed to live long. When I asked Mr. Gasanov from Russia what rules he had for living a long life, he said, "I did not know I was going to live 153 years, so I don't have rules." Here we have a perfect answer—one that shows that the mind and the body are intact. He just went along without being affected by the factors that break down the body.

We have to realize that through philosophy and our mental faculties, we see that people are different. In the study of man, you find we are not all calcium types, we can't all be long-lived people, we can't all live in that perfect climate. Some of us want to live with our families even if they live at the North Pole or at the equator. There are people who are interested in building and in doing things that can be done only in a certain climate. Some people are engrossed in government, clubs, communities, some in armies, and some are working with machines and doing things that are just unbelievable; and it takes successful people to do certain things that are demanded of them in civilization today. We have to recognize types of people and the study of Brominosis, which is the study of man. I can't put it any better than the old sage when he said, "Know thyself."

If it weren't for the different mental faculties, the different feelings within the soul itself to either migrate, to change the position, to live with certain people, or to get out of a certain place where you aren't happy, then we would not have the variety of accomplishments today. It takes a certain type of person to design an airplane. We have to have innate abilities to build houses, structures, edifices, forts, conservatories, observatories, factories, even pyramids. We can't all be happy and satisfied just living a long life, plowing in the fields and feeling that this is all there is to live by. The greatest thing we see in all of this is that a *long life lived is not good enough, but a good life lived is long enough.*

Some people lean towards the spiritual centers while others do not. There are some people who have a feeling for the rules of wisdom and an obedience to a divine self. They feel a power within them, and they feel a power on the outside that is greater than themselves.

They recognize that there is such a thing as "lip-service" to religion and praise that is not good or sincere. They

dislike hypocrisy of every type and will not tolerate quack-
ery. These people admire honesty, virtue, integrity; it
makes them strong in honor. These people become enthusiastic about sages of the past, about their books and
teachings. Many times they are interested in changing
conditions that seem not right to them and may even be
considered fanatical by others who may think they have
gone to extremes, not realizing that each person thinks a
little bit differently.

Some, by developing their spiritual faculties, turn
against the old world and want to see it end in order to
bring in the new world. There are some who go so far as to
think that the mind is everything and forget the physical
body. They become over-enthusiastic about metaphysics,
modernism, spiritualism, fairy tales, hypnotism, psy-
chism, new creeds, experimenting with new thoughts,
going into new discoveries, dreams and the interpretation
of dreams. Anything that is unknown or extraordinary,
interests them and they even go into the unseen worlds.
Many of these people are prone to exaggeration and will
build up the extraordinary and the mystical phenomena.
They may go so far as to develop the psychic centers,
become interested in psychic phenomena and the spirit
world. Others who have entirely different spiritual
centers, may try to expose them, and then there is con-
flict.

The elderly people I met do not go to such extremes. I
am convinced it is because they are of a calcium type,
down to earth, balanced; they are not mental people and
you find they are not inventive. They are not going off into
the mental realms so much that they forget their physical
bodies. Their day is well-balanced—physically, mentally,
and spiritually.

I have studied for many years and I recognize that some
people want health, and they are going to try to get it by
any means. While we are talking about philosophy which
includes love, the spiritual side of life—what we are studying, peace and harmony—we find that the word "health"
came from the old Teutonic language which meant salvation. It is our salvation.

If good health is our salvation, how do we get it? We
get it from being natural, pure and whole. This doesn't
mean just eating whole rice, it means a whole man physically, mentally and spiritually. I do feel that while so

many today are praying for health, this is only one part. My mother used to say that health was not everything, but without health, everything else was nothing. So today, it shouldn't be a matter of just praying for money. This is only part of what you should have. We need even more than just peace and harmony. Why not pray for God's will to be done, rather than our own. I think that we should be ready for whatever is yet to come, but I feel that what we should pray for most is knowledge. We need knowledge. We perish for a lack of knowledge. We need wisdom. We need a wise domain to live in. And above all things, we need guidance. These are the three things we should pray for, and then we will have a good life, and we will have as long a life as we are supposed to have. We will go through life doing the things that I am sure God will approve of.

Above all, you should be living a spiritual life, which is Number One as far as I am concerned, and then, second, a good mental life, and third, the physical. The physical without the mind will run amuck. You will never accomplish or do anything which God would approve of, outside of just existing, repairing and rebuilding. That would be what we call a low order in life. But man was created above all animal life and in the image of God. This is the spiritual accomplishment in life.

I feel this, that you could have all the physical things you want, but if there is no love in your heart, then I think it amounts to nothing. I think, too, that if you don't have any happiness, what's the use of living? I mean, what is it without some friends around you? These are mental things, but they are more spiritual than anything else. These are the things that make for a balanced life, and I found most of the old men had them.

Los Angeles Herald-Examiner, Thursday, March 6, 1975

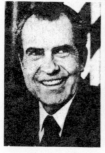 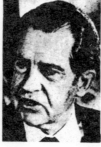

Political events and a near-fatal illness have taken their toll on Richard M. Nixon. Photos show him in 1973, above left, at his farewell last August and, at right, last November after 23-day stay in Long Beach Memorial Hospital.

Just to live for physical purposes only is no good. This includes a house, for a house is never a home until you have somebody you love within it and flowers around it. Until then, you've just got four walls. You need something on the inside of that house, something warm and inviting to your friends—a cheerful kitchen, relaxing furniture, windows to let in the sunshine.

We need to get along with each other mentally, and we need to find a way for us all to live together spiritually in a way that our physical bodies can accomplish and perform necessary activities in agriculture, building, etc., in order to unify our lives. I could go on still further. I would say that soul growth is most important of all for developing the higher nature of man. I believe the inner man is most important to take care of.

From here on, individual growth comes in, and you find that what a man is intrinsically, that is what he really is. Soul growth is important to our inner self and our progress in the eternal struggle. I think that everybody likes to be *somebody* in this life. Everybody wants to be wanted—we should live so that we are wanted and are loved.

The elderly people have a good philosophy. They believe nobleness and a good character are two of the great things that they should follow through with in life. Having a noble background and having a noble parentage was very important to them. Humility was also very important. They recognize that everyone should have his say. One person talks and everybody listens. Another person starts to say something, no one will interrupt. No one. They listen. They have the patience to listen until others are finished.

Purity is another important trait. They recognize pure joy. They find joy in simple things: in flowers, in their soil, with their animals. It is something to recognize. Most of society today has to have joy through stimulation and through excessive motivation. We can't take the simple things and find the pure joy that goes along with them.

The joy center of the mind is something that has to be fed in everyone. We have to have that little triumphant feeling that comes through cheering activities. The elderly people live in rapture and just swell up in joy. We, too, can become unusually happy in this kind of joyous activity. In most of these elderly people we find the joy center of the brain is well developed. They are not the "heady" type, and are not so jubilant that they are constantly jumping for joy, because they are of the calcium type. They are well grounded on the earth, but they appreciate all the good that is around them. When people are joyous and enter into that feeling, they do not carry around gloom and despair.

They feel they have to be worthy of what they are doing. You even have to be loveworthy, you have to be worth your love. They are thinking deeply of love. They practice love. They say that love should be worked out in their feelings. Who works love out in their feelings? I have a *feeling* of love for you. We find that happiness and joy is very important to them. They must have happy moments. They don't want to leave you until they know you are happy. When they once know you, they throw their arms around you to give you their complete self and to let you know they have a warm, loving feeling for you. It is a great feeling to have somebody kiss you and to know they haven't something like Alka Seltzer in their mouth. It's really something to have them throw their arms around you and know they mean it. It is important to go through life and have feelings expressed as they should be expressed.

They also reckon kindness to be one of the greatest qualities a person could possess. They strive to be kind to one another.

One of the great things we find in these people is that they don't know they are doing the unusual thing. For instance, I asked Mr. Gasanov if he ever had a doctor. "No," he said, "I never had a doctor." "Did you ever take any pills?" "No." "Did you ever have constipation?" "What is that?" he asked. "Well," I explained, "do your bowels move every day?" "Why certainly, doesn't everybody's?" He didn't know that people's bowels don't move. I asked him about his diet. "Diet, what do you mean by diet? I live on all the fruits and vegetables of the area and I eat them when they come in."

These elderly people have lived with the soil, the natural environment. They lived in perfect hygiene because of the altitude. In the Hunza valley the people live practically the same as they did in the lowlands. The water in the lowlands, however, is not as hygienically pure as in the highlands. The sunshine destroyed bacteria that wasn't destroyed in the lowlands. Heat developed bacteria that you didn't get in the highlands. They were living in an environment that was entirely different.

Some people are introverts and prefer being by themselves. Some people live a greedy existence. But you never really recognize this greedy existence until you travel around and see what other people are like. You should go to Europe and then when you return to America you will see how tips are almost demanded wherever you go. It is part of a national greed, I am convinced. I believe it. I don't believe in tips. I feel we should be kind and good to people without being bribed. I learned something from one of the horse trainers that was here. When I gave some sugar and carrots to my little colt to come to me, he said, "Never bribe a horse. You want that horse to come up to you because he loves you."

In this country, we have so much turmoil and resentment, resistance and confusion. We have expectations that always lead us to disappointments which are hard on the nerves and hard on the mind. This is the kind of life we live

One of the greatest Keys we have I learned from a man who lived 256 years. His name was Li Ching Yun, from the Szechuan province of China, and he died in 1933. He was a man who gathered herbs—long-life herbs such as ginseng, gotu kola and fo tsi tung. He gathered all of these for years and used them daily. It was part of his life. He claimed at age 90 he cut down his life a great deal because he played tennis too hard. This man tells you to sit like a dog and run like a tortoise, to rest and not overdo.

I wondered just what it was that gave him his long life. Was it the bark from trees that he gathered? Was it the sap from bushes; was it the herbs in the field? Then I wondered just what do you want to do in life? Do you want to be a mechanical automaton that just exists? Is the mind most important? What do we do as we go through life? Are bowel movements everything? A good heartbeat? Imagine marrying a person for just this, and no more.

This is not enough. We have to put all of these qualities together and find a full, good life. I believe that the example of all these things put together will help to give you this long life, good life, healthy life to the very end. This old Chinese man was asked before he died to what he attributed his long life and he gave us one of the greatest Keys, when he said, "I attribute my long life to inward calm."

I would like to say that I didn't find that *all* of the old men lived *all* of the Keys perfectly; but I do believe those who lived the longest and healthiest lives were those who practiced the use of these Keys in their daily lives. Some of these people weren't aware of the things they were doing because they were living such a natural life that God was just taking care of them, and they didn't know what was happening. It is nice to be in a place where you don't even know what is going on, and yet you're still doing the right thing.

We have traveled and seen how all these people live; yet it is very difficult to get this into our own way of living. A lot of these things are not easy to do in civilization. Some of them you are not going to be able to do because you are married. Some of them you are not going to be able to do because you have to make money. You've got a job and an apartment or house to take care of. You might be living around a lot of noise. You might be living near a radio station that has its evil effects from a radiation standpoint. Or, you might be living around some nuclear plant and you have radiation to consider. You could be living someplace where the cold weather is so harsh that·you can't get warm enough on a lettuce leaf to exist. It's hard to be a vegetarian in the north. If you are going to be a good vegetarian, you should be where there are tropical foods and tropical weather. I mean, that goes with it. Many of us can't get this together in one place.

I still, however, come back to this one thing I mentioned in the very beginning. It isn't just living a long life that counts, but have health enough so you don't live in pain. I have never met a perfectly healthy person. There is no such thing. The healthy person doesn't exist. Most of us are free from pain and are not constipated, but that doesn't mean you are well. If you can live your life and die as natural a death as possible, I think this is what we should work for. This is the only reason to have any good health at all, so we don't have to retire before we die. We can work until we die. I think having good health in the last part of our life is something more of us should think about. You can do this only by trying to prevent disease and living in a more natural environment. This would be in the country where trees are, and in a good altitude.

FRIENDSHIP

Friendship is very important, in fact it is invaluable. Joy is also invaluable when we realize what happens in the body. The nervous system has to qualify feeling. The word "emotion" comes from "e", meaning ego, and "motion", meaning move. "I move", that's what we do. We move to the situation. Do you know what worry means? Look it up sometime. Worry means to choke. And it does! If you have worry on your mind, you are going to have to change. You have life in order to enjoy life. It is no good to think that because we have *things,* we have a better life. If you have the outside *things* and are trying to fix up your inside, that's working backwards! You must start from *inside.* Don't give your attention to the thing that is choking you. Worry is faith working in reverse. Worry is concentrating on something you don't want. Replace worry with something good. As soon as you do this, all other things will become right.

The nerves are what I have to take care of today; yet all the fasting experiments (and we have a lot of scientific tests of fasting) show that the nerves never degenerate and break down in fasting. You can degenerate all the muscle structures and the fat and the bones, but the nerves will never break down. They hold on until the last.

When nerves cause heart trouble, it is because the driver is like a nervous chauffeur. You have a good heart, but how do you drive it? Have you been holding the reins too tightly. Have you been giving them good thoughts? Where is your dwelling place? Where do you abide?

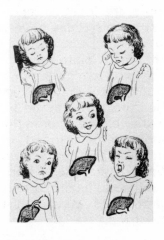

Conclusion

I have traveled far and wide over the years. I have visited many countries and found that the people in these various countries have cultures which have been passed along to them, through their inheritance and through their ancestors, up to the present.

I was able to see these people in dance; I was able to see them in counsel; I was able to see them in court; I was able to see the physical and mental, and the spiritual elements all at work. I went into their churches; I was interested in their philosophy. I might add that the elderly person offered me the greatest opportunity of all to learn. I did not get the counsel here that I got from the elderly. I found that the wisdom of the ages is the wisdom of the sages. I learned that the fool does not know what is in the wise man's head, but the wise man knows what is in the fool's head because he was once a fool himself.

I looked into their great hearts and had an insight into the minds of these men. I know that the wise man is not born, but is made. I was able to see the levels of consciousness that exist in a man who has lived a long time. I don't think that any of us have lived long enough to give this world the wisdom it needs or desires.

Our young people are looking for a better world in which to live. Most people today have experienced sicknesses and are looking for a way out. So to those who are seeking their youth, or striving to keep it, may I say I hope you realize that when you reach for it or touch it, it can be quite an elusive thing; for it may not be in just an active body or a good heartbeat; it may be in that moment of thankfulness for a life well spent, or in the love that comes to you from a good wife, or husband, or your grandchildren. It may even be in the appreciation of a beautiful sunset. But whatever it may be, I hope your youth includes happiness and good health, a long life with friends and a short one on troubles. May you touch this youth at any and every age of life.

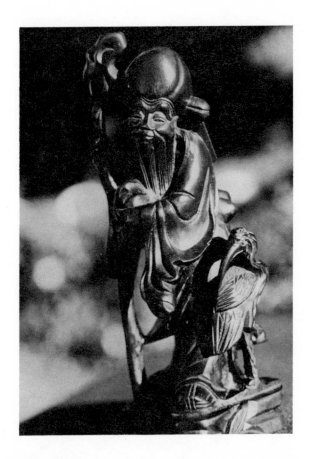

No, this is not the end. This can be the dawn of a new day. May health and long life begin with you.